CW00542034

HERBAL ANTIBIOTICS

Tips and Tricks to Make Effective Herbal Antibiotics to Cure Daily Common Ailments

SHARON BICKEL

© Copyright 2023 - All rights reserved.

The content contained within this book may not be reproduced, duplicated, or transmitted without direct written permission from the author or the publisher.

Under no circumstances will any blame or legal responsibility be held against the publisher, or author, for any damages, reparation, or monetary loss due to the information contained within this book, either directly or indirectly.

Legal Notice:

This book is copyright protected. It is only for personal use. You cannot amend, distribute, sell, use, quote or paraphrase any part, or the content within this book, without the consent of the author or publisher.

Disclaimer Notice:

Please note the information contained within this document is for educational and entertainment purposes only. All effort has been executed to present accurate, up to date, reliable, complete information. No warranties of any kind are declared or implied. Readers acknowledge that the author is not engaging in the rendering of legal, financial, medical, or professional advice. The content within this book has been derived from various sources. Please consult a licensed professional before attempting any techniques outlined in this book.

By reading this document, the reader agrees that under no circumstances is the author responsible for any losses, direct or indirect, that are incurred as a result of the use of information contained within this document, including, but not limited to, errors, omissions, or inaccuracies.

Table of Contents

Introduction

Have you ever felt like you had some sort of infection but weren't sure what it was? Maybe you tried taking over-the-counter medications, and they didn't work. If this sounds familiar, then it may be time to explore herbal antibiotics as part of your healthcare routine.

Herbal antibiotics are gaining popularity as many people realize that natural treatments can be just as effective, if not more so when it comes to treating common illnesses. Herbs such as lemon balm, garlic, and ginger have been shown to possess powerful antibiotic properties, allowing them to be used in place of commonly prescribed medication. This is especially useful for those who don't want to use pharmaceutically-made drugs for whatever reason.

When traditional medications fail to treat an ailment or condition, herbs can often provide some relief. Many people find that herbs can be very effective without leading to undesirable side effects that are typically associated with typical medications and treatments. The best part is that herbs don't often interact with other forms of treatment or medication, reducing any potential risks involved. Even though natural therapies like herbal remedies have been around for centuries, modern medical science has not yet incorporated them on a large scale, but this may soon change as we continue to discover the incredible health benefits they provide.

Knowing how to make effective herbal antibiotics is one of the most useful skills anyone can have. It can be used not only to treat minor ailments naturally but also for emergencies where time or access to prescription drugs is limited. While it takes some knowledge and practice to master the craft, almost anyone can learn it with some research and instruction. This guidebook will help you along the way by providing all the basics needed to make your herbal antibiotics.

We'll start by discussing exactly systemic, non-systemic, and synergist antibiotics, so you can understand the different types of medicinal properties found in herbs. Next, we'll show you how to set up your herb lab so you have all the necessary supplies for making herbal remedies. Then, we'll provide some essential safety tips and tricks for handling and storing your herbs as well as harvesting them from nature if needed. After that, we'll get into the real fun stuff - the herbal medicine-making handbook. Here you'll find detailed instructions on how to make your herbal antibiotics for headaches, common ailments, and even digestion problems.

Regardless of the kind of problem you're facing, learning to make your herbal antibiotics can be an invaluable skill that has lifelong benefits. We hope this guide will serve as a helpful resource for you as you explore the world of natural healing and take control of your health. Good luck and happy healing!

Chapter 1

Systemic Antibiotics

Antibiotics have become a major tool in modern medicine due to their proficiency in fighting bacterial infections. Overuse of antibiotics has been rampant in the last few years, leading to antibiotic resistance and a growing problem. However, many illnesses can be defeated without the use of antibiotics, for example, drinking plenty of fluids, getting lots of rest and exercise, and eating healthy foods. In addition, antibiotics should be taken as directed by your doctor or healthcare professional. Doing so not only ensures that you successfully recover from illness but also helps protect us from the emergence of antibiotic-resistant bacteria.

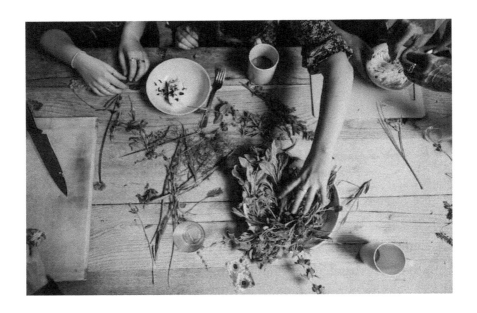

But what if natural alternatives could be used in place of antibiotics? Natural remedies can relieve symptoms and ward off bacterial infections without the side effects of antibiotics. In this chapter, we will discuss systemic antibiotics, their common uses, the ailments they treat, and a list of herbal alternatives that can be used in place of antibiotics. The herbs and ingredients on the list will be discussed in detail, including their source, description, and antibacterial properties. So, let's get started!

Systemic Antibiotics

Systemic antibiotics are essential to modern health care, often used to treat bacterial infections. These powerful drugs are administered either orally or intravenously and absorbed into the bloodstream to target and kill or stop the growth of invading bacteria. However, as with any pharmaceutical drug, incorrect dosage or overuse can cause health problems and antibiotic resistance. Because of this, proper monitoring of systemic antibiotic usage is vital for effective treatment compared to other methods, such as topical creams and ointments, when combating certain infections. Patients should always consult their physician when considering treatment plans with systemic antibiotics so that the best use can be made from these useful medications.

Common Uses

Systemic antibiotics are generally used to treat bacterial infections, such as wound and urinary tract infections. They work by directly killing the bacteria in the body or preventing them from reproducing. In more serious cases, they may also be used as part of a combination treatment involving multiple medications. Systemic antibiotics can also be taken before medical procedures to prevent infection. For instance, these medications may be prescribed before surgery to reduce the risk of postoperative complications. They can even be given prophylactically during pregnancy if signs of infections are present to help protect both mother and child from potential harm. Here are some common uses for systemic antibiotics:

1. Skin Infections

Systemic antibiotics can be used to battle skin infections when topical treatments are not effective. Examples of infections that may require systemic antibiotics include impetigo, cellulitis, and MRSA. The specific antibiotic prescribed for each infection varies depending on its cause, severity, and other factors. The most commonly prescribed systemic antibiotics for skin infections include amoxicillin, clindamycin, and ciprofloxacin. These medications have the potential to reduce inflammation, prevent bacterial growth, and eradicate existing bacteria.

2. Urinary Tract Infections (UTI)

Urinary tract infections (UTIs) are very common, especially among women. One of the primary ways that UTIs are treated is with systemic antibiotics. Systemic antibiotics work throughout the entire body to help clear up the infection quickly and effectively. Most UTIs will respond to appropriate antibiotic treatment within a couple of days, although some may require longer courses of medication. Unfortunately, many people are concerned about the long-term effects of taking antibiotics frequently or in large doses and their impact on overall health. It is crucial to follow your doctor's advice when it comes to treating UTIs, as this is ultimately in your best interest.

3. Respiratory Infections

By the millions, people endure respiratory infections annually. This is a pervasive issue that should not be overlooked. Although antibiotics are often the first course of treatment to deal with such infections, systemic antibiotics should only be used in severe cases. Medical practitioners must assess each case individually, taking into account the known background data and symptoms before prescribing systemic antibiotics. Overutilization of these drugs can reduce their effectiveness while treating infection and cause serious side effects ranging from nausea, vomiting, and diarrhea to more long-term issues such as increased levels of antibiotic resistance and impairment of the microbiota existing inside our bodies. Ultimately, it is critical to understand the takeaways associated with carefully deciding when these systemic antibiotics should be prescribed and taken.

4. Sexually Transmitted Infections (STI)

Systemic antibiotics such as doxycycline and azithromycin are the most commonly prescribed to treat various sexually transmitted infections or STIs. While these systemic antibiotics can effectively rid an individual of an active STI, they cannot necessarily prevent a person from contracting one in the future. It is crucial to take other steps for maximum protection, such as always using barrier protection when engaging in intercourse and being tested regularly for bacteria or viruses that can cause STIs. Even individuals who consider themselves "low risk" should still be tested annually to ensure they remain free of infection.

5. Gastrointestinal Infections

Bacterial gastrointestinal infections often lead to debilitating symptoms, negatively impacting a person's quality of life. Systemic antibiotics are commonly used to treat gastrointestinal infections, as they help disrupt the growth of bacterial cells and can reduce symptoms in a matter of days. Unfortunately, widespread use of systemic antibiotics can lead to antibiotic resistance and decreased effectiveness over time. Therefore, individuals should consult with their doctor before using these medications to ensure that the prescribed antibiotic is tailored to their specific infection and likely to provide results.

6. Bronchitis

Bronchitis is a common respiratory infection caused by inflammation of the mucous membrane in the bronchi. It's a contagious condition that can be mild or severe and sometimes can linger on, turning into a prolonged chronic ailment. The most commonly prescribed treatment for bronchitis is the systemic administration of antibiotics. These drugs reduce and eliminate symptoms quickly and safely by targeting infection-causing bacteria. In some cases, corticosteroids are also prescribed to prevent any potential or developing complications, such as exacerbations or airway obstruction. Doctor check-ups should be scheduled regularly when undergoing treatment with systemic antibiotics to monitor any possible side effects or altered responses.

7. Pneumonia

Pneumonia is an ailment that causes difficulty breathing and is common in the young, elderly, and immunocompromised. Because of this, it is especially crucial to protect against and treat it quickly. In most cases, pneumonia can be treated with antibiotic medications taken orally or intravenously. These systemic antibiotics work to attack the infection directly, stopping the spread of the bacterium or virus which caused pneumonia. Depending on its severity, symptoms may persist for days or weeks. However, continued use of antibiotics during this time will help prevent complications that could lead to long-term pulmonary disorders or even death.

8. Bladder Infections

Bladder infections can be an excruciatingly painful experience, often making even the simplest acts of sitting and moving around uncomfortable. These infections result from bacteria entering the urinary tract, can make you feel rundown and feverish, and come with a potent base urine odor. Fortunately for those afflicted with bladder infections, relief can be obtained through systemic antibiotics that fight infection-causing agents and clear up the infection within a few days. However, if left untreated, a bladder infection can potentially develop into a kidney infection requiring more intensive medical attention. Therefore, take immediate action when symptoms of a bladder infection are noticed to combat the ailment effectively and avoid complications.

9. Kidney Infections

Kidney infections are a serious but often preventable health concern. Systemic antibiotics have been proven to effectively treat such infections by eliminating bacterial growth that can cause urinary tract issues and result in damage or failure of the kidneys. While self-care, such as hydration and good hygiene habits, can reduce the risk of kidney infections. Consulting with a medical professional should be done at the first sign of infection symptoms, including pain in the sides or lower back area, abnormal urine odor and color changes, fever, chills, and nausea. Early diagnosis and treatment are essential for avoiding further complications from an infection.

10. Pelvic Inflammatory Disease (PID)

Pelvic Inflammatory Disease (PID) is a serious and potentially life-threatening condition caused by an infection in a woman's reproductive organs. Symptoms, which can range from mild to severe, include pelvic or abdominal pain, fever, chills, irregular menstrual bleeding, vaginal discharge, and painful urination. With proper medical treatment and care, PID can be effectively treated with systemic antibiotics, thereby reducing the risk of long-lasting complications such as infertility, chronic pelvic pain, and ectopic pregnancy. Early diagnosis is crucial to quickly manage the ailment and end its progression before it causes permanent damage to the internal organs. Unfortunately, due to a lack of awareness, many women do not realize they have PID until it is too late. Therefore, regular check-ups for all women should be encouraged for proper detection and timely treatment of Pelvic Inflammatory Disease.

Natural Alternatives

Systemic antibiotics are a crucial part of treating severe infections but can be detrimental to our bodies and the environment if overused or misused. Thankfully, natural alternatives to systemic antibiotics are emerging that both effectively treat illness and reduce some of the risks associated with traditional antibiotics. These alternatives include probiotics, herbal teas, honey, and garlic -all of which may not be able to take the place of systemic antibiotics in serious cases, yet they have proven to provide relief from lesser infections. We must investigate various plant-based methods as an additional remedy to existing antibiotics as we strive for healthier and more sustainable solutions for fighting illnesses.

1. Goldenseal

Goldenseal, also known as Hydrastis Canadensis, is an herbal medicinal plant native to the eastern United States and Canada. It is part of a family of plants called Ranunculaceae, and the root of goldenseal has been used in traditional medicine for centuries. In more recent times, goldenseal has been found to have antibacterial properties which help treat mild skin infections and overall immune system strength. Goldenseal's active ingredient, berberine, may even be effective against multi-drug-resistant bacteria and fungal infections. Altogether, its numerous benefits make it sought after among natural health enthusiasts worldwide.

2. Echinacea

Echinacea is a flowering herb used in traditional medicine for centuries. Belonging to the daisy family, indigenous Americans first used it for aiding the immune system and treating ailments such as colds and flu-like symptoms. The active ingredients of echinacea are believed to fight off bacteria and viruses, helping boost a person's immunity. Although available in capsule form from pharmacies, some argue that wild harvesting its medicinal properties can be even more beneficial by providing more concentrated levels of nutrients. With research into this remarkable herb still ongoing, we cannot wait to find out what other uses echinacea has!

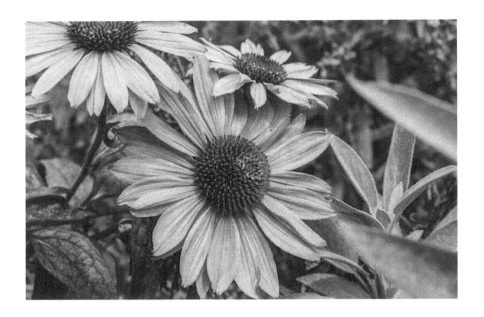

3. Ginger Root

Ginger root is an iconic part of many traditional cuisines, originating from South Asia and China. Today, several varieties of ginger are being produced worldwide, most notably in India and Nigeria. Many people are familiar with eating ginger raw or cooked in a meal, but it has recently become a popular ingredient used to make tea due to its many benefits. Scientifically, ginger root is known for its strong antibacterial properties that effectively protect against illnesses. It comes in many forms, including dried powder, freshly grated root, or capsuled extract. You can find these from any local market or grocery store, and make sure you are stocking up on this amazing immunity-boosting ingredient!

4. Garlic

Garlic is an incredibly versatile and flavorful ingredient that can be found in many different types of cooking. The pungent and distinctive flavor of garlic imparts a delicious aroma to whatever dish it is added to, whether it is a pasta dish, roasted vegetables, salad dressing, or even spread on toast with butter. Additionally, garlic has long been appreciated for its antibacterial properties; ancient Egyptians believed in garlic's ability to protect them against illness and disease. Today, scientific studies have proven that garlic possesses natural antimicrobial properties; regularly consuming garlic can help fight infection, reduce inflammation, and improve digestion.

5. Oregano Oil

Oregano oil is one of the most potent natural remedies available today. Derived from wild oregano plants, the essential oil packs quite a punch when it comes to fighting bacteria. Oregano oil contains two powerful agents, carvacrol and thymol, that are responsible for their extraordinary antibacterial properties. Studies show that oregano oil can be used to treat skin conditions, thyroid issues, fungal infections, and even certain forms of cancer. While it is most commonly used for therapeutic purposes in supplement form, you can also add oregano oil directly to food as a flavoring agent or an aromatherapy diffuser as an environmental disinfectant. Whatever your purpose, oregano oil might be the answer to your medical woes.

6. Turmeric

Turmeric is a historical and flavorful spice used in many Asian cultures. It has a deep, almost burnt orange color, and its flavor hints at ginger, pepper, and turpentine. Derived from India, where it has been used since ancient times to treat everything from depression to heartburn. Nowadays, turmeric is being cultivated all around the world for its high antibacterial properties. Recent studies have indicated its efficacy in clearing up stomach issues such as indigestion and ulcers, as well as its potential for providing relief from joint pain. The versatility of turmeric makes it an incredibly useful ingredient for many delicious dishes and health supplements used for thousands of years.

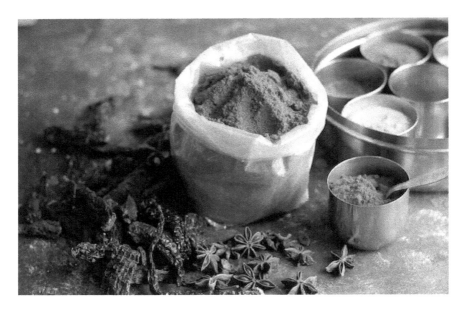

7. Manuka Honey

Manuka Honey is a special type of honey produced by bees in New Zealand who use the nectar found in the Manuka tree flowers. It has strong antibacterial properties that make it a highly sought-after ingredient in the medical and health industry. Manuka Honey can be used both topically and internally due to its remarkable healing power, which scientists attribute to Methylglyoxal, a compound found naturally within it. It has a wide range of applications, from reducing skin inflammation to healing wounds and combatting bacterial infections. Manuka Honey is also known for its distinctive taste. It has a higher sugar content than regular honey but with a unique, earthy flavor profile. There are many beneficial attributes associated with this special type of honey that makes it essential for natural health solutions.

8. Tea Tree Oil

Tea Tree Oil is an essential oil that is derived from Melaleuca Alternifolia, a species of tree native to Australia. Distillation of the leaves and twigs yields an oil with strong antibacterial properties, making it an ideal treatment for certain types of skin infections. Tea Tree Oil has long been used as an herbal remedy by indigenous Australians, and it can still be found today in many home pantries and bathroom cabinets as a natural remedy for acne, cuts, scrapes, and various other skin conditions due to its multiple medicinal applications.

9. Neem

Neem, or Azadirachta indica, is a tree native to India and Myanmar and is now cultivated in tropical climates worldwide. Known for its many medicinal uses and antibacterial properties, this evergreen tree has been integral to Ayurvedic healing practices for centuries. Parts of the neem tree, such as its leaves, bark, and oil, are commonly used not only in traditional medicine but also in cosmetics, soaps, shampoos, detergents, and in agricultural pest-management treatments. The unique antibacterial activity of neem is due to the balance of triterpenoid compounds found within it; these compounds can be effective against bacteria on both the skin's surface and within deeper layers. There is even potential for using neem-based creams or gels to treat certain types of bacterial infections.

10. Holy Basil

Holy basil, or tulsi, is a herb from India that has long been used in the country's holistic system of health and healing. It was traditionally known as "The Incomparable One," and today, it is seen as a natural remedy for numerous physical and mental health ailments. Its leaves have a distinct aroma which can be attributed to its high concentration of active compounds, such as eugenol and ursolic acid. Not only are these components beneficial to the human body, but they also possess antibacterial properties that can help fight off infection-causing bacteria on the skin or lining of the stomach. Holy basil has become an increasingly popular supplement over recent years due to its ability to provide natural relief without any potential side effects.

11. Cabbage

Cabbage is a hardy, cool-season vegetable that is rich in dietary fiber, vitamin C, and antioxidants. It is an excellent source of minerals such as manganese, potassium, calcium, and magnesium. This versatile vegetable can be eaten raw or cooked and can also be used to make sauerkraut. Not only does cabbage provide nutrition and flavor to our diet, but it also has potent antibacterial properties that help fight off infections. Researchers have found that eating cabbage or drinking a cup of cabbage juice a few times a week could give us protection against certain illnesses. So next time you are looking for something juicy and nutritious to add to your diet, why not try some fresh crunchy cabbage?

12. Pau d'arco

Pau d'arco is an herbal remedy found in the rainforest areas of South America. It is known for its antiviral, anti-inflammatory, and antibacterial properties due to compounds with antioxidant and anti-cancer activities that are present in its bark. Recently it has been gaining interest for its potential as a natural treatment for various microbial infections. The research on Pau d'arco is still ongoing to further explore the numerous therapeutic uses this herb may have. Due to possible gastrointestinal side effects such as nausea and abdominal pain, it is crucial to take it under the guidance of a healthcare professional if one decides to try this herbal remedy.

Systemic antibiotics, when used properly, can be a helpful remedy for many of the ailments that plague us. From bacterial infections and strep throat to respiratory issues and more, these drugs have been used effectively to combat a variety of problems. Not only are they relatively easy to obtain and administer, but the momentary discomfort associated with them is well worth the long-term outcome in most cases. With responsible use and following physician-prescribed dosages, systemic antibiotics can be an effective and prudent way to treat or manage certain conditions.

Chapter 2

Non-Systemic Antibiotics

Non-systemic antibiotics are a powerful but commonly used medication to fight off bacterial infections. These drugs work by infiltrating the inner workings of foreign bacteria and breaking down the cell walls. This allows the body's natural response to eliminate any remaining bacteria and viruses that could be causing harm. Non-systemic antibiotics should only be used for specific infections and for a short period to prevent developing antimicrobial resistance.

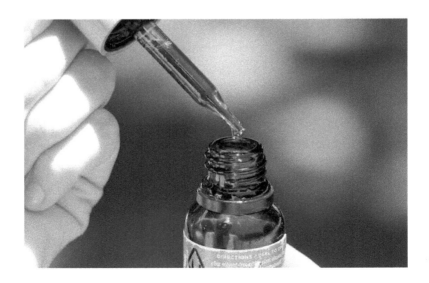

Research by the World Health Organization has shown that non-systemic antibiotics are incredibly effective, helping millions around the world to combat all types of bacterial infections with ease and leading to happier, healthier lives. In this chapter, we will discuss non-systemic antibiotics, their possible applications, and some natural remedies that can be used instead of conventional treatments. From honey to pepper, read on to find out what natural antibiotics can do for your health. This can be an invaluable resource for those looking to take a more holistic approach to their healthcare.

Non-Systemic Antibiotics

Non-systemic antibiotics are topical medications that can be applied directly to the site of infection, as opposed to being taken orally or injected. This form of treatment has many benefits and can be effective in treating localized infections such as pink eye, acne, ear infections, and skin lesions. Unlike systemic antibiotics, there is no buildup of antibiotic resistance when using non-systemic medications, making them safer and more effective over the long term.

Non-systemic antibiotics have been used to treat bacterial infections since the 1940s. They usually take effect quickly after being applied and remain effective for a short period, often referred to as a "half-life." They are most frequently used in the treatment of common dermatological conditions such as acne, impetigo, and infections of the feet, hands, and nails.

Additionally, these types of antibiotics can be beneficial for treating mild systemic infections if administered early before it has become too severe. This is especially vital in preventing ailments from becoming more serious due to an increasingly ineffective response from the body's natural defenses. Non-systemic antibiotics offer quick relief from stubborn bacteria without causing any significant side effects when used properly.

The side effects associated with non-systemic antibiotics tend to be much milder compared to oral or injection treatments, and they can reduce the risk of certain illnesses spreading further. In conclusion, non-systemic antibiotics are an incredibly useful form of medication that can effectively treat a variety of irritating illnesses without the need for high doses or single-exposure therapies.

Common Ailments Helped

Non-systemic antibiotics can improve conditions like respiratory infections, earaches, urinary tract infections, sore throats, and even some skin irritations like impetigo or cellulitis. By completely killing off the infection-causing bacteria in localized areas of the body, non-systemic antibiotics can rapidly reduce symptoms and minimize the potential for serious complications. Non-systemic antibiotics are also typically far better tolerated than their systemic counterparts. They're easy to administer, don't generally lead to unintended side effects on other systems or organs in the body, and also don't require extended courses of medication. Doctors, therefore, almost always opt to use non-systemic antibiotics first unless there is clear evidence that a disseminated type of infection has taken hold.

1. Infections

Non-systemic antibiotics are a powerful tool in the fight against infections. These medications work especially effective against localized areas of infection like ear, eye, skin, and upper respiratory infections. Non-systemic antibiotics also reduce antibiotic resistance because they only attack specific bacteria associated with particular infections and don't disturb beneficial bacteria that play a crucial role in maintaining health. For these reasons and more, non-systemic antibiotics have become an increasingly popular choice for treating bacterial infections.

2. Inflammation

Inflammation is an essential part of the body's healing process. However, when it is unwanted or occurs too frequently, it becomes a cause for concern. The good news is that non-systemic antibiotics designed to target the specific strain of bacteria causing the problem can manage inflammation. Non-systemic antibiotics block the growth and spread of bad bacteria while leaving good bacteria in place, reducing inflammation and its associated symptoms. Not only do they serve to alleviate short-term discomfort and irritation, but they also help patients remain healthy long term. All in all, non-systemic antibiotics provide a safe and effective means of managing chronic inflammation and its related issues.

3. Stomach Aches

Stomach aches can feel like the last thing you want to deal with, especially when it's a chronic issue. Thankfully, certain antibiotics can help ease some of these uncomfortable stomach issues. Non-systemic antibiotics specifically target the infection in your intestines without affecting your entire body system. This means they don't have as many side effects that can come with other medicines. In essence, this antibiotic acts like mortar which binds and seals the wall of bacteria in your intestines so that the infection cannot spread, thereby allowing you to begin feeling better quickly. Talk to your doctor today to figure out if non-systemic antibiotics are right for you and your situation. Together, you can make the right choice to get on the road towards relieving your painful stomach aches at last.

4. Cold And Flu Symptoms

There are antibiotics available that don't just treat bacterial infections but can also be used to alleviate the symptoms of colds and flu. These non-systemic antibiotics attack only the specific area the medication is applied to, which could bring relief from sore throats, congestion, and coughing and even reduce the fever associated with either illness. While always best to talk to a healthcare professional before administering any kind of medication for cold or flu symptoms, non-systemic antibiotics can be an invaluable aid during this time of year!

5. Allergies

Allergies can be an incredibly frustrating and debilitating condition, but recent research has demonstrated that non-systemic antibiotics have the potential to significantly lessen those symptoms. Non-systemic antibiotics are delivered externally to the skin, and they work by helping the body develop a kind of "tolerance" against common allergens like dust and pollen. In studies, people with a wide range of allergies have shown positive results, making this therapy a potential game-changer for allergy sufferers all over the world. Non-systemic antibiotics promise to provide quick relief without the associated risks of other treatments, such as cortisone injections or systemic antibiotics. As research continues, it looks increasingly likely that this form of treatment could revolutionize how millions of people must live with the daily challenges their allergies cause them.

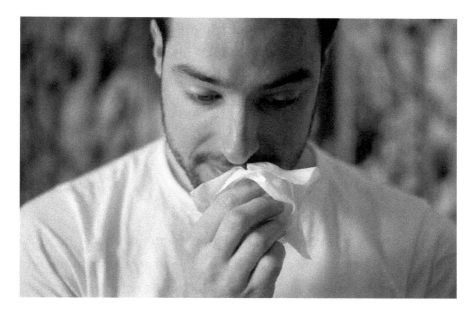

6. Skin Irritations

Skin irritations can be incredibly annoying and uncomfortable, especially when left untreated. Fortunately, non-systemic antibiotics can help treat a wide range of skin problems, from pimples to eczema. Some of these antibiotics can be applied topically directly to the skin, while others are meant to be taken orally. Topical creams and ointments that contain non-systemic antibiotics can help reduce inflammation, redness, and itching that accompany skin irritations.

In addition, oral medications containing non-systemic antibiotics can help reduce the skin's oiliness and promote healing.

7. Respiratory Problems

The use of non-systemic antibiotics can greatly impact respiratory problems. When a doctor prescribes non-systemic antibiotics to an individual, it typically means they target infection at the site where it is localized. For instance, if there is fluid buildup in a single lung, this medication can work to neutralize the bacteria causing the infection and limit the further spread of infection through respiration. Furthermore, these types of medications tend to have fewer side effects than systemic antibiotics because they remain within the specific area offering relief from symptoms such as breathlessness and chest pain.

8. Eye Irritations

When it comes to treating eye irritations, antibiotics can provide great relief. When eyes become inflamed due to an allergy, a foreign object, or an eye infection, topical antibiotics can help get rid of any bacteria present in the affected area and reduce the level of inflammation. People with existing health issues should not use non-systemic antibiotics because they may interact adversely with their medications. Taking advice from a doctor before using non-systemic treatments should always be your first course of action!

9. Ear Infections

For those with ear infections, antibiotics are often the first course of treatment. However, it's not always necessary to take systemic antibiotics. Non-systemic antibiotics can reduce the number of bacteria in the middle ear without affecting other parts of the body. These medications work quickly and may provide some relief from both pain and discomfort within a few days. While non-systemic antibiotics can be largely effective for treating ear infections in many cases, follow-up visits to your physician are crucial to ensure that any irritation has cleared up and that serious complications have not developed as a result of infection.

10. Mouth Sores

Non-systemic antibiotics are a form of treatment for mouth sores that are not caused by systemic infections. Generally, these antibiotics will contain active ingredients that have anti-inflammatory, antibacterial, and other properties, which can help to reduce pain, swelling, and irritation associated with mouth sores. If necessary, they can also be used in conjunction with other treatments, including over-the-counter medications, supplements, or dietary changes. When choosing an antibiotic, it is crucial to consult a doctor to ensure that it is appropriate for the type of sore being treated.

Natural Antibiotics

Natural alternatives have become increasingly popular as more people become aware of the health risks of taking non-systemic antibiotics. Companies have begun offering natural supplements and formulas that offer relief from the symptoms of bacterial infections. These remedies often include herbal extracts, medicinal mushrooms, and probiotics for gut health. Some natural alternatives can reduce inflammation in addition to alleviating infection symptoms. These alternatives are less prone to provoke side effects than pharmaceutical antibiotics and promote natural body functions with added nutrients and minerals. Ultimately, natural alternatives to non-systemic antibiotics provide safe and effective treatments for a variety of issues.

1. Honey

Honey is a remarkable substance used by many cultures throughout history to treat physical and mental ailments. It is a naturally occurring sugar syrup produced by bees from the nectar of flowers and secretions from other insects such as scale insects. In addition to being highly nutritious and valued for its antibacterial and antifungal properties, honey offers numerous health benefits. It has been known to help boost immunity, aid in weight loss, reduce inflammation, and treat allergies. Furthermore, because it is so sweet tasting, many people use it in recipes or opt for it as an alternative to white sugar or artificial sweeteners. All in all, honey is truly a superfood with tremendous potential when consumed or applied to skin or hair.

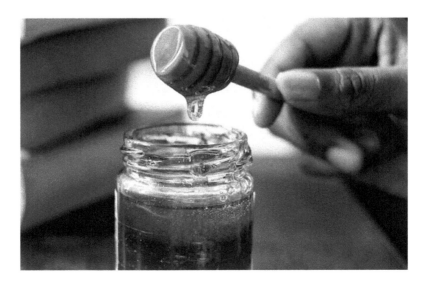

2.   Cinnamon

Cinnamon is an aromatic spice derived from the inner bark of certain tree species from the genus Cinnamomum. The most common sources of cinnamon come from Ceylon, Indonesia, and Vietnam. Cinnamon has a rich history. It was used by ancient Egyptian physicians to treat coughing and other respiratory issues since the 22nd century BC. Though a popular cooking ingredient, cinnamon also offers some surprising health benefits. It is a natural anti-inflammatory and is often used to reduce swelling and bloating in the body. It also contains anti-diabetic properties, which can help control blood sugar levels naturally to fight against diabetes. Additionally, Cinnamon helps improve circulation by increasing blood flow which is key for healthy skin and hair growth, as well as aiding muscle recovery after workouts.

3.   Coconut Oil

Coconut oil has become a household essential for many individuals looking for an all-natural cure-all. Referred to as a 'superfood' in some circles, this unique oil can be used for cooking various types of food, treating the skin and hair, and even fighting off diseases. Typically derived from the meat of mature coconuts, it is known for its high levels of medium-chain fatty acids that contain antibiotic and antioxidant properties, making it more beneficial than other oils. People often take advantage of its high nutritional qualities by using it as a dietary supplement or topical ointment to gain relief from conditions such as eczema, psoriasis, or other skin irritations. To sum up, coconut oil has risen in popularity thanks to its wide range of applications, both edible and medicinal, making it an invaluable addition to any home.

4. Apple Cider Vinegar

Apple cider vinegar is an incredibly versatile and medicinal food that can be consumed and applied in a variety of ways. It is produced from apples that have been cut, crushed, and fermented. The result is a potent liquid rich in essential acids, enzymes, vitamins, and minerals that are thought to provide beneficial health effects. The wide range of apple cider vinegar benefits includes helping to regulate blood sugar levels, aiding digestion, improving heart health, boosting the immune system, supporting weight loss efforts, and much more. Easily obtainable in most grocery stores or health food retailers, it's easy to integrate this all-natural remedy into one's diet or regular beauty regimen.

5. Myrrh

Myrrh is aromatic and medicinal incense used in many cultures for thousands of years. A potentially-sacred substance, it was one of the gifts presented to baby Jesus by the Three Wise Men. It has a unique, slightly bitter aroma, and many refer to it as an oleo-gum resin that comes from small trees and plants native to parts of Africa, Arabia, India, and Yemen. When burned or placed on hot charcoal, its health benefits have been said to include increased respiratory health, improved digestion, cognitive clarity, energy levels, and even wound healing. In addition to being used medicinally throughout history and in various rituals today, myrrh is also believed to be associated with protection against negative energies.

6. Thyme

Thyme is an aromatic herb with a lot of culinary and medicinal uses. It's a member of the mint family and is an easy-to-grow perennial plant. The leaves and flowers of Thyme are the sources from which this herb can be used. Despite its small size, it packs a big health punch when consumed in the form of tea or added to food as an ingredient. Its flavor adds a unique taste to dishes, and its high antioxidant properties help reduce inflammation, maintain immunity, and lower cholesterol levels for a healthier body.

7. Clove

Clove is a popular spice renowned for its unique sweet, slightly pungent aroma and complex flavor. It is obtained from the unopened flower buds of a tree scientifically known as Syzygium aromaticum. Clove has been used in traditional medicine around the world for centuries, and recent scientific studies have validated many of its health benefits. It contains properties that act as an antioxidant, antifungal, and antimicrobial, which help support digestion and reduce inflammation in the body. Studies conducted on animals have also found that it may possess gastroprotective benefits due to its inhibition of gastric acid secretion. Furthermore, clove oil has proven to be effective against dental pain and potentially helpful in oral care. All in all, clove is more than just a flavorful condiment; it is also an ingredient with therapeutic potential that goes beyond taste enhancement.

8. Pepper

Peppers are a ubiquitous ingredient in various global cuisines, adding flavor and pungency to make dishes truly stand out. The spice can come from a variety of sources, most commonly the Capsicum family of plants, which includes chili peppers of all varieties and colors. Pepper is an incredibly healthy spice, offering numerous benefits ranging from reduced risk of metabolic syndrome and heart disease to fighting inflammation with antioxidants. While the exact health properties vary based on the particular type of pepper used, all are linked to improved health outcomes when consumed regularly. Whether used for flavor or nutrition, or both, peppers are sure to enhance any dish or recipe.

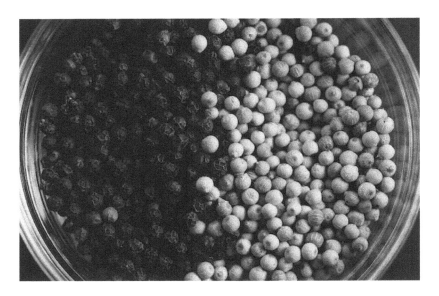

9. Lemongrass

Lemongrass is an aromatic plant used to flavor food and drinks as well as for its purported health benefits. Most commonly found in

Southeast Asia, lemongrass also grows in subtropical climates around the world. The health benefits associated with lemongrass include improving digestion, curbing inflammation, battling bacteria, and providing antioxidants. It even relaxes the body and mind. For optimal use of the full potential of the herb's holistic healing powers, it can be consumed as a tea or a supplement while also being used in cooking or fragrance products as an energy-boosting ingredient. Whether brewed into tea or sautéed in stir-fry dishes, lemongrass is packed with nutrients and provides an intense flavor profile that cooks around the globe have loved for centuries.

10. Grapefruit Seed Extract

The grapefruit seed extract is gaining in popularity as a supplement due to its many health benefits. It is derived from the juice and pulp of grapefruit seeds and contains natural antiviral, antibacterial, and antifungal compounds. Those who want to reap its rewards can purchase it in liquid or capsule form at most natural health stores or online retailers. A grapefruit seed extract has been found to boost immunity, fight yeast infections, reduce inflammation, aid in digestion, and prevent illness. While more research is needed on the best doses and uses of this supplement, there appears to be a place for it in anyone's health regime.

11. Anise

Anise, also known as Aniseed, is an aromatic herb that belongs to the Apiaceae plant family. It has a licorice-like flavor and sweet aroma, widely used for cooking, liqueurs, and medicinal purposes. Anise can grow either by direct sowing of the seed or transplanted and watered on a regular basis in order to flourish. Some of its benefits include helping with digestive issues such as indigestion and flatulence, aiding with respiratory illnesses like bronchitis, boosting the immune system, and detoxifying the body. Additionally, the seeds are said to possess anti-inflammatory properties, which could help alleviate joint pains from conditions like arthritis. According to ancient medical texts, it contains high levels of antioxidants which help improve overall health. Anise can be found in various forms, such as powder, oil extracts, essential oils, and distillations accessible online or at local grocery stores or specialty shops.

Non-systemic antibiotics are commonly used to treat infections, inflammation, and other ailments. While pharmaceuticals have their place, there may also be natural alternatives that can provide relief and health benefits without the side effects of drugs. Herbs like garlic, turmeric, oregano oil, clove, pepper, lemongrass, and grapefruit seed extract are all-natural ingredients that have antibacterial, antiviral, antifungal, and other medicinal properties. While research is still ongoing to determine the full health benefits of these items, it is crucial to be aware of their potential and understand how they can be utilized to improve overall well-being. Regardless of one's lifestyle and diet, these ingredients can offer health benefits suitable for anyone's needs.

Chapter 3

Synergist Antibiotics

Antibiotics have been used to treat bacterial infections for many years, but as microbial resistance increases, a new approach is needed to overcome this issue. Synergist antibiotics have become an essential tool in the medical arsenal against bacterial infections. Synergist antibiotics are safe and effective, making them powerful allies in the fight against antibiotic resistance and providing new hope for those suffering from bacterial infections.

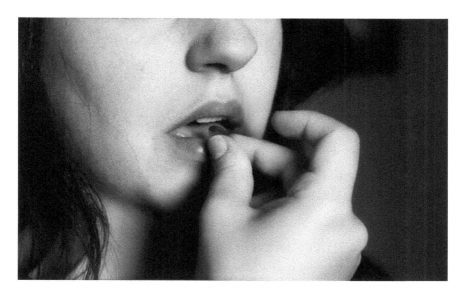

Although antibiotics are often used to treat bacterial infections, they can also have adverse effects when taken in large doses or for long periods. This chapter will discuss the definition of a synergist antibiotic, its mechanism of action, clinical uses, adverse effects and contraindications, and its benefits. It will also explore the different types of synergist antibiotics and their natural alternatives. By understanding these concepts, we can better use synergist antibiotics and natural alternatives to promote health and well-being.

Definition of Synergist Antibiotics

Synergist antibiotics are a class of drugs used to help combat difficult-to-treat bacterial infections. Usually, they are combined with other types of antibiotic treatments, such as tetracyclines or penicillin. The addition of these drugs helps boost the effectiveness of antibiotic therapy and increases its ability to target and eliminate the infection. Synergist antibiotics combine two or more separate drugs to enhance the patient's therapeutic effect. The synergy of two or more drugs enables doctors to gain better control over these diseases with fewer doses and shorter treatment courses, reducing the amount of time the bacteria have to develop resistance to the drugs.

Synergist antibiotics make it harder for bacteria to resist the action of antibiotics, which makes it easier for the medication to work its way throughout the body and eliminate any remaining bacteria. Synergistic antibiotics are vital for treating bacterial infections that have become resistant to commonly used antibiotics, and their use could prove to be a key factor in keeping drug-resistant infections from spreading further. The use of synergist antibiotics also helps reduce the amount of drug-resistant bacteria in the environment.

Mechanism of Action

Synergist antibiotics play a vital role in treating serious bacterial infections. Their mechanism of action involves blocking the bacterial cell from synthesizing certain proteins, which then prevents the bacteria from growing or dividing. A synergist antibiotic is most effective when combined with other antibiotics as its mode of blocking protein synthesis is different from other types of antibiotics. When used together, the synergistic effect between the two antibiotics can result in a greater effect on killing and preventing the growth of bacteria than either type alone. This makes it a powerful tool for fighting serious infections and providing relief to patients.

Clinical Uses

Synergist antibiotics are among the most powerful weapons in a medical professional's arsenal when it comes to tackling antibiotic-resistant infections. This type of antibiotic drug combination works by inhibiting different steps of bacterial cell wall synthesis, which allows them to be more effective against bacteria that otherwise may be resistant to single antibiotics. Synergist antibiotics also have proven benefits beyond simply combating infection. They can reduce certain bacteria's ability to form biofilms which further reduces the likelihood of an infection forming or persisting and helps limit the spread of infection within a facility. In addition, they can allow for lower concentrations of any given antibiotic and therefore minimize potential side effects from those drugs. Synergist antibiotics are the go-to choice for many healthcare professionals in tackling serious and drug-resistant bacterial infections.

Adverse Effects and Contraindications

Synergist antibiotics are a valuable tool in treating certain bacterial infections; however, their use can have adverse effects and contraindications. Side effects can include diarrhea, stomach cramps, nausea, headache, and rashes. Furthermore, those suffering from pre-existing conditions or allergies should abstain from using this antibiotic. Those taking anti-inflammatory medications such as aspirin may experience additional gastrointestinal issues when using synergist antibiotics. To diminish patient risk and increase effectiveness, the treating physician and the patient must be aware of any contraindications before initiating treatment with this antibiotic.

Benefits of Synergist Antibiotics

Synergist antibiotics create a stronger treatment than a single antibiotic would. Synergist antibiotics can be used as primary treatments, reducing the need for high-strength single antibiotics that are more likely to lead to resistance. They also limit side effects and reduce the amount of medication required to cure bacterial infections, making it easier and less costly for patients to recover. Synergist antibiotics can also be tailored specifically for each patient, helping ensure they receive the exact treatment they need while minimizing drug interactions. Here are some more benefits of synergist antibiotics:

- Improved effectiveness against antibiotic-resistant bacteria

- Faster resolution of infection with fewer complications

- Lower risk of side effects and drug interactions

- Reduced drug concentrations, allowing for better control of infections without increasing the risk of resistance.

- Fewer side effects due to lower drug doses

- More targeted treatments tailored to the patient

- Increased accuracy of medications tailored to each patient

- Cost-effective treatments

Types of Synergist Antibiotics

Synergist antibiotics are used in treating complex infections or when bacteria have become resistant to other antibiotics. The two main types of synergist antibiotics are synergic and combinatorial, each with its unique benefits. Synergetic antibiotics involve two medications that act together in fighting an infection and which are often prescribed together for maximum effectiveness. Combinatorial antibiotics involve three or more medications and can alter the genetic makeup of bacteria so that it is less likely to become resistant to treatment. Both types can be very effective in eradicating infection and preventing recurrence in the future.

A. Penicillin

Penicillin is a type of synergist antibiotic that is effective in treating a wide variety of bacterial infections. This natural antibiotic, derived from molds, works to inhibit the growth of bacteria by destroying their cell walls. In addition to being an effective treatment for illnesses caused by bacteria, it has almost no side effects and rarely causes an allergic reaction. Penicillin is also highly cost-effective compared to other antibiotics, making it one of the most commonly prescribed antibiotics worldwide. It is used both to treat acute infections as well as for long-term preventative treatments, and its success proves why penicillin continues to be relied upon for its tremendous healing power decades after being discovered.

B. Cephalosporin

Cephalosporin is a type of synergist antibiotic made from a group of naturally occurring compounds known as beta-lactam antibiotics. Cephalosporin has been used for decades and is recognized for its incredibly high efficacy in fighting infections. It works by preventing the bacteria from forming the walls that will protect them, thereby killing the bacteria before they can cause any harm to the body. Interestingly enough, due to its expansive effects on different types of bacteria, cephalosporin is sometimes even labeled a "super antibiotic." While taking over-the-counter medications may seem like an easy solution when fighting an infection, investing in cephalosporin's powerful antibacterial properties might just be the best defense against more severe illnesses.

C. Amoxicillin/Clavulanic Acid

Amoxicillin/Clavulanic Acid is one of the most powerful antibiotics available, which can treat multi-drug-resistant bacteria. This synergist antibiotic works by inhibiting certain enzymes called beta-lactamases found within bacterial cell walls and that normally break down beta-lactam antibiotics, such as amoxicillin.

Amoxicillin/Clavulanic Acid is often prescribed for severe infections where regular antibiotics cannot be used. It has been an especially valuable tool in treating acute and chronic diseases. In addition to its antibiotic properties, this combination has anti-inflammatory properties, making it even more effective in treating infections caused by bacteria. Overall, Amoxicillin/Clavulanic Acid is a safe, efficient, and invaluable antibiotic with the potential to cure various bacterial infections.

D. Carbapenem

Carbapenem is a type of synergist antibiotic that is used to treat severe infections and take control of life-threatening gram-negative bacteria and even dangerous multi-drug resistant bacteria. It inhibits the production of cell walls in such organisms, which leads to the disruption of their growth. In contrast to other forms of antibiotics, carbapenem is impervious to stressors like acids, bases, and dehydration which makes it preferable over other conventional treatments. Despite their reliability, carbapenems should always be used as a last resort because prolonged use tends to contribute to increasing drug resistance as well as emerging new serious types of infections due to certain recently identified strains against which carbapenems may not be effective at all.

E. Monobactam

Monobactam antibiotics are a type of synergist that is typically used as part of more comprehensive treatments to combat serious infections. This is because monobactams do not affect many Gram-positive organisms but act effectively against many different kinds of Gram-negative ones. When used in combination, other antibiotics may enter bacterial cells more easily and add to the efficacy of treatment, thus creating an environment in which it is difficult for pathogens to survive or resist the effects of medication. Monobactams can either be broad-spectrum or specific, and they are powerful, with few serious side effects, when used correctly in prescribed doses. Their use can help restore balance to a disrupted internal system while providing some protection from dangerous diseases and illnesses.

F. Aminoglycoside

Aminoglycosides are potent synergist antibiotics developed to fight a wide range of bacterial illnesses, from pneumonia and bronchitis to sore throats and ear infections. Developed in the 1940s, these antibiotics have remained a cornerstone treatment for bacterial infections. Aminoglycosides work by interfering with the bacterial cell wall and inhibiting protein production, leading to the destruction of the bacteria.

While their effectiveness is undeniable, aminoglycoside toxicity can cause kidney damage when administered in large doses or for prolonged periods. In addition, these drugs should not be used without first determining that the bacteria responded sufficiently to other antibiotic treatments, as they may further contribute to drug-resistant bacteria if used incorrectly. Despite this risk, aminoglycoside antibiotics remain essential to many doctors' arsenals in treating pernicious bacterial illnesses.

Natural Alternatives to Synergist Antibiotics

Natural alternatives to synergist antibiotics are becoming increasingly popular due to the emergence of antibiotic-resistant bacterial strains. By exploring nature's medicine cabinet, there may be a way of developing safe and effective drugs that don't carry the risk of resistance or severe side effects. Some of the most promising compounds include compounds derived from honey, garlic, oregano, and even citrus peel.

Research is ongoing to determine how these natural remedies can work in concert with existing antibiotics as an additional tool for healthcare professionals to provide better quality care for patients. Results so far have been encouraging, with some showing a dramatic decrease in bacteria populations when using these combinations compared to using traditional treatments alone. With the rising prevalence of antibiotic resistance worldwide, finding cost-effective and sustainable treatments could make all the difference.

A. Herbal Medicine

Herbal medicine is often seen as a natural alternative to antibiotics and other medications. It typically involves using herbs, plants, and other natural ingredients to relieve illness or disease. Herbal medicines are most commonly taken in the form of tinctures, capsules, or teas. Herbs can be used topically and orally through oils, creams, compresses, and gargles.

Herbal medicines have the potential to be combined with antibiotics to create a synergistic effect that will expedite healing and provide more effective results than either could accomplish individually.

These properties may help reduce the risk of developing antibiotic resistance in some cases. Much research has been conducted on how herbal remedies interact with antibiotics to improve their effectiveness while reducing side effects compared to antibiotics alone. As such, many people are looking at natural alternatives in the hope of finding safer and more efficient treatments for various ailments.

B. Essential Oils

Essential oils have become a popular natural alternative to traditional antibiotics due to their ability to safely fight bacteria and virus infections. Research has shown that essential oils help balance the microbiome, supporting the body's natural defense system while minimizing any side effects that traditional medications can bring. They also contain active compounds capable of enhancing the therapeutic effect of synergist antibiotics, allowing for long-term treatment effects with minimal risk. Essential oils are best used in combination with other treatments, such as probiotics or dietary changes, to create a more holistic approach to healing illnesses and maintaining health. This approach allows consumers to achieve a better quality of life without relying too heavily on costly prescriptions.

C. Probiotics

With the increasing concern of traditional antibiotics becoming less effective due to overuse, probiotics may just be the solution we are looking for. Probiotics are living microorganisms that provide health benefits when consumed in adequate amounts, and research has shown that they can effectively replace or be used as a complement to traditional antibiotics. Moreover, probiotics help restore healthy microbiome balance in the body and improve digestive health, immunity, and overall well-being. This makes them a natural alternative with no side effects to traditional antibiotics and provides long-term therapeutic benefits.

D. Diet and Nutrition

With spring just around the corner, many are looking to cleanse and detox using natural methods such as diet and nutrition. Natural antibiotics can be effective in providing defense against bacteria without harsh chemical components that can upset the balance of our internal environment. Combining two antibiotics to combat more intense illnesses, synergist antibiotics have become increasingly popular, particularly with the introduction of various natural alternatives.

Foods like honey, garlic, and onions offer high antibacterial properties, while probiotics such as yogurt, miso soup, and kimchi can provide support for good gastrointestinal health. In addition to foods, herbs such as Echinacea, ginseng, and oregano oil are known for their immune-boosting effects when taken internally. While dietary choices may not treat or cure any serious illnesses, the power of natural ingredients shouldn't be overlooked when supporting our overall wellness.

E. Homeopathy

Homeopathy is becoming an increasingly popular form of alternative medicine, as it offers a natural alternative to synergist antibiotics.

Homeopathic treatments rely on specific doses of diluted ingredients to balance the body and cause the body to respond by relieving the symptoms. Homeopathy is effective for acute and chronic illnesses, including allergies, digestive issues, headaches, flu-like symptoms, and depression.

The best part is that there are virtually no side effects when taking homeopathic remedies, unlike conventional medications, which may lead to unpleasant side effects like drowsiness or weakened immunity. Furthermore, since homeopathy works in harmony with your body's natural capacity to heal itself, it causes only minimal disruption to the overall balance of your health. Homeopathy may be just what you need if you're looking for a natural solution that won't wear down your immune system over time.

F. Exercise and Stress Reduction

The current trend in health and wellness is to seek natural alternatives for achieving and maintaining good physical health, and exercise is a great way to do that. Our bodies were designed to be active, and regular physical activity greatly benefits both your body and mind. When it comes to stress reduction, exercise can be a powerful remedy. Exercise releases endorphins, the hormones that help enhance your mood and make you feel happier naturally. You don't need expensive drugs or therapies when you have access to the great outdoors right at your fingertips! Here's an easy way to get yourself moving - try taking a brisk walk every day. Be sure to find time in your schedule to devote some physical activity, as this will improve your physical well-being and reduce your stress levels significantly.

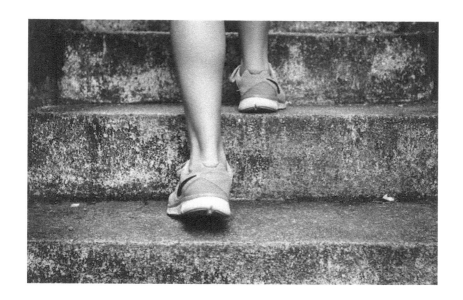

G. Aromatherapy

Aromatherapy is a natural, non-invasive alternative to fighting infection and preventing the spread of bacteria with antibiotics. Essential oils provide a holistic approach to treating an array of health issues, from congestion to skin infections. Rather than fishing for a prescribed chemical solution, which can often cause unwanted side effects and overuse, aromatherapy works much like plants in nature. Achieving balance internally unlocks the body's natural healing capabilities, allowing it to heal and restore itself. By optimizing the ratio of individual essential oils for each therapeutic purpose, we can clear out the mess inside our bodies and bring ourselves into synchronization with the environment outside. Aromatherapy may not replace standard medical treatment, but it should certainly be considered as part of an overall plan for good health and well-being.

H. Probiotics

Probiotics are becoming more popular as a natural alternative to antibiotics. While antibiotics treat the symptoms of an infection, probiotics are meant to maintain balance in the gut microbiome, strengthening the body's natural defenses and helping it fight off illness. Probiotics can also be taken with antibiotics, reducing the overall side effects of antibiotic use. Taking a daily probiotic supplement is one way of preventing infections while keeping the microbiome balanced. Probiotics have been shown to reduce inflammation and improve digestion, both of which can raise immunity against infections. With research continuing on their benefits, probiotics could be a great solution for those looking for a strong immune system without having to rely on drugs.

I. Spices

Spices are a natural alternative to synergist antibiotics, offering an effective form of treatment for bacterial infections. As spices have evolved and been used throughout history, they've developed unique characteristics that possess anti-microbial properties found to fight bacteria. Current studies have shown that compounds such as clove oil demonstrate incredibly effective antifungal and antimicrobial qualities. Unlike antibiotics, many of these compounds can be consumed in large enough quantities to effectively treat bacterial infections without the risk of damage to beneficial bacteria living in the stomach, skin, and gut. Furthermore, spices also offer a greater variety than antibiotics for treating conditions without producing resistance, giving them a distinct advantage over traditional treatments.

Given the dangers of antibiotic resistance, there is a growing demand for natural alternatives to antibiotics. Several herbal treatments and ingredients can be used as natural antibiotics and are often just as effective, if not more so, than traditional medicines. Whether it's aromatherapy, probiotics, spices, or herbal compounds such as garlic, these natural treatments offer a safe and effective way to treat common bacterial infections without the risk of antibiotic resistance. With this in mind, it's worth exploring these natural remedies before resorting to traditional antibiotics. Your health will thank you for it.

Chapter 4

Building Your Herb Lab

Herbs and plants have been utilized since ancient times throughout the world for their healing properties, playing an essential role in many cultures. They have been used as a natural approach to treating physical ailments without the need for pharmaceutical drugs. Herbal remedies are still relied on and commonly used today, ranging from teas and tinctures to homemade salves and even powders. Many natural products support the body's systems, helping it to find balance. Some herbs can be taken for specific needs, such as supporting digestion, relieving congestion, or providing antioxidants and vitamins to help invigorate the body holistically.

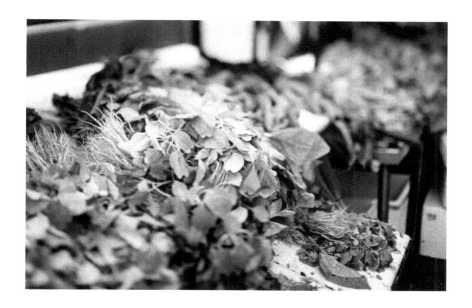

Whenever possible, herbal remedies can be an advantageous choice for everyday health. Today, an increasing number of people are turning to herbalism as a way to take control of their health and well-being. With the help of a well-stocked herb garden and an understanding of herbs, people can now create their own medicine in the comfort of their own homes. This chapter will explore the benefits of having an herb garden, how to start growing one, and the necessary tools needed to build a functioning herb lab. The tips and tricks section will offer helpful advice when it comes to growing and harvesting herbs, as well as provide insight into some popular herb varieties that can be planted.

Benefits of the Herb Garden

Having an herb garden can be incredibly beneficial for a variety of reasons. Fresh herbs have more flavor and aroma than the dried varieties found in traditional grocery stores, offering much more unique flavor profiles to any dish. An herb garden provides easy access to ingredients needed for home-cooked meals, reduces store trips, and saves time and money. When cooks grow their herbs, they also get to choose exactly what type of organic gardening methods they want to use. Herbs are also useful for medicinal purposes as well as cooking, offering natural remedies that can help people maintain their well-being with fewer chemicals. In addition, herbs offer homeowners a variety of beautiful plants that bring life and vitality to gardens or backyards while helping them breathe easier outdoors by promoting clean air circulation.

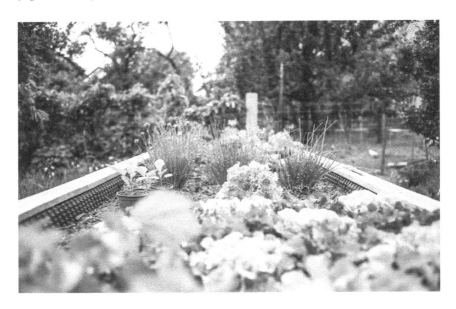

1. Fresh Herbs

One of the primary benefits of having an herb garden is that you will always have fresh herbs on hand. Herbs can be used to add flavor to a variety of dishes, and they are also a great way to add some extra nutrition to your diet.

2. Save Money

Another benefit of having an herb garden is that it can save you money in the long run. Herbs can be expensive to buy at the grocery store, but if you grow them yourself, you can get them for a fraction of the cost.

3. Know What's in Your Herbs

When you grow your herbs, you will know exactly what is in them and how they were grown. This is essential because many store-bought herbs may contain pesticides or other harmful chemicals.

4. Improve Your Health

Herbs can also be used to improve your health in a variety of ways. For example, basil improves digestion and relieves stress, while rosemary boosts cognitive function and memory.

5. Attract Wildlife

An herb garden can also be a great way to attract wildlife to your yard or garden. Birds, bees, and butterflies are all attracted to the flowers and scents of herbs, which can provide them with a valuable food source.

6. Enhance Your Home's Curb Appeal

An herb garden can also enhance your home's curb appeal by adding color and interest to your landscaping. Herb gardens can be designed to fit any space, whether it's a small plot in your backyard or a large bed in your front yard.

7. Improve Your Soil Quality

Growing an herb garden can also help to improve the quality of your soil over time. As the herbs grow, they will release nutrients into the soil that will help other plants grow better. Additionally, using organic gardening methods will help improve your soil's overall quality.

8. Connect with Nature

Spending time tending to your herb garden can also be a great way to connect with nature and get some fresh air. Gardening has numerous mental and physical health benefits, so it's a great activity to do for both your body and mind.

Growing Your Herb Garden

An herb garden can make a world of difference in your life. You're getting the freshest and most flavorful ingredients by growing your herbs. Plus, tending to an herb garden is a therapeutic activity that can be done indoors or out. It doesn't take an expansive plot of land either, as some herbs, such as basil and parsley, can thrive even for apartment gardening in containers. Many herbs are also perennials that come back year after year with minimal care. Growing an herb garden can be a fun, rewarding experience that is sure to please the senses. In the next section, we'll explore finding the right space for your garden and preparing the soil for planting.

Finding Space for Your Garden

Creating a place for an herb garden can be challenging in the midst of everyday life, especially if you live in a small home or apartment.

Fortunately, there are plenty of creative solutions available to maximize whatever space you may have. From vertical planters or herb walls to hanging window boxes or balcony gardens, let your imagination and resourcefulness take charge! When creating your herb garden, make sure to take into consideration sunlight exposure and water access. Additionally, the kinds of herbs you select should depend on your desired use for them, whether it be preparing an appetizing dish or utilizing their medicinal value. Whether it's indoors or outdoors, gardening has many advantages and can bring great satisfaction when done correctly.

A. Indoor vs. Outdoor Growing

Discovering the ideal environment for growing your herb garden can be challenging. Deciding between indoor and outdoor growing each has its benefits, from improving air quality to ensuring plant security. Turning an area of the home into an indoor herb sanctuary can prove to be the perfect solution for those who do not have a lot of outdoor space to work with. With the right lighting and proper environmental control, you can create a thriving habitat for your herbs that is easy to manage and requires minimal maintenance. Whether deciding on indoor or outdoor cultivation, taking the time to prepare will ensure your plants are healthy and successful as they enter their life cycle.

B. Access to Sunlight

While gardening offers a wonderful feeling of accomplishment, achieving optimal growth in your herbs requires sunshine. Finding space for your herb garden can be the most challenging part, but it's worth taking the time to make sure they have adequate access to sunlight. Since they need 8-10 hours of direct light every day, find a location close to windows or outdoors that will provide them with plenty of warmth and illumination. If growing indoors, it may be necessary to supplement natural light with other sources, such as grow lights multiple times daily, to ensure proper sunlight exposure. Once you've identified a sunny spot for your plants, you're ready to get busy and enjoy the rewards of this fun and fulfilling experience!

C. Identifying the Best Location for a Garden

If you're searching for the perfect spot to plant your herb garden, start by considering access to sunlight. Herbs thrive in areas with direct exposure to six or more hours of sun daily. You'll also need some level of protection from strong winds as this can dry out plants in a matter of hours. Once these two criteria are met, take into account its placement with other plants within your garden. Most herbs prefer well-draining soil and dislike their roots sitting in water, so it's crucial to include a raised bed if you live in an area with frequent rainy days. It's also critical to think about how practical picking and snipping branches might be. Choose a spot close enough so movement won't be too inconvenient and weeds will be easier to remove without damaging anything else. After all, bases are covered; it's time to enjoy the fruits of your labor!

Preparing the Soil

For anyone looking to get their hands dirty and start an herb garden, preparing the soil is critical to your success. Whether you're a seasoned green thumb or new to the gardening game, giving your herbs a good foundation with suitable soil is essential. First, remove any weeds and break apart any lumps of dirt with a spade or rake. Be sure to mix in compost or peat moss to help create heavier, nutrient-rich soil. To ensure proper aeration of the ground and further promote plant growth, use clean sand used for masonry work and slowly hoe it in. Be careful not to compact the dirt too much. With that done, you'll have the perfect foundation to cultivate your garden.

A. pH Balance

One of the most important considerations when it comes to soil preparation is ensuring that the pH balance is correct. pH stands for "potential of hydrogen" and describes the level of acidity or alkalinity in soil, which can have major implications on nutrient availability, water penetration rates, and overall plant health. Depending on the type of herbs you plan to grow, you will have different needs, but ranges should typically fall within 6.5 to 7.2 pH for optimal growing conditions. Fortunately, there are many natural ways to adjust pH if it is not already within this range, such as with Sulphur or lime applications, meaning you can achieve perfectly balanced soil without relying on harsh chemicals.

B. Fertilizing

The best way to ensure vibrant and healthy growth is by fertilizing your soil with a well-balanced mix of organic materials. Investing in high-quality compost or manure will give your plants the essential macro and micronutrients they need to thrive. A slow-release fertilizer is also recommended, as it can help maintain optimum nutrient levels over a longer period. Additionally, you should ensure that your soil has good drainage so that excess water doesn't get stuck around the roots. Preparing your soil properly with fertilizers and good aeration means strong, healthy plants that require less maintenance in the long run.

C. Mulching

A key part of that groundwork is mulching. Mulch can limit weeds, moderate temperature extremes, and conserve water. It also protects plant roots from temperature extremes and helps add nutrients to the soil over time. Various materials make suitable mulch, such as bark chips, grass clippings, leaves, compost, and pine needles. For optimal results, spread whatever material you choose two to three inches deep across the exposed soil in your herb garden. Keep in mind that different types of mulches require different levels of maintenance throughout the season, so check out how often each needs to be replenished or replaced before you select one for your herb garden.

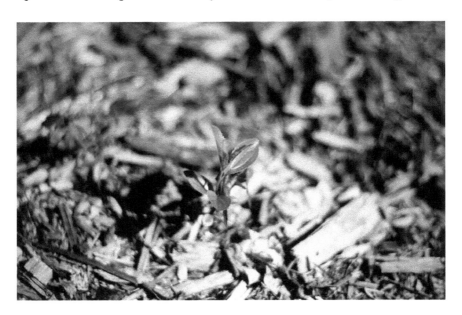

Necessary Tools and Supplies

Starting your herb garden is a rewarding experience that will yield beautiful results. To ensure you get the most out of your gardening experience, however, it's crucial to have the right tools and supplies.

A. Garden Tools

Before planting the first seedling, stock up on high-quality soil, soil amendments, fertilizers specifically tailored for herbs, individual pots or a raised-bed planter box, hand pruners, and shears (for keeping plants neatly trimmed), watering cans or hoses of different sizes (to suit small and large plants respectively), a rake or hoe for digging holes and general cleanup, gloves for protection when handling plants or soil, and stakes or trellises for supporting climbing plants. With these essential supplies on hand, you'll give your herb garden the care it needs to produce healthy greens throughout the growing season.

B. Containers

Whether you want to spruce up your balcony, start a patio garden, or can't commit to taking care of a large outdoor herb garden, starting an herb garden in containers is an excellent way to get started. Containers can be as small as tomato-sized pots or decorative planter boxes. The benefit of planting herbs in containers is that it gives you control over soil composition and moisture levels, which will help ensure the success of your plants. Herbs are incredibly hardy, thriving in almost any kind of container, making them the perfect choice for novice gardeners. Start by picking a few varieties that match the conditions of your space and are suitable for container gardening, then just add water, some fertilizer, and lots of love!

C. Irrigation Supplies

Growing an herb garden is a rewarding experience. With the right supplies, proper care, and a little bit of patience, you can have your supply of fresh herbs all summer long. Irrigation supplies are crucial to keeping your herb garden healthy and productive. Investing in the right amount of water and soil nutrients will ensure that your herbs get what they need to grow and thrive. Consider adding a drip irrigation system or water timers to ensure each plant gets the right amount. Too much or too little water can be detrimental to their health. Also, provide slow-release fertilizer throughout the growing season for optimal results!

D. Lab Equipment

If you're looking to make your herb garden the envy of your gardening friends, some lab equipment can ensure the best results. Lab spoons and scoops allow for precision when collecting the exact amounts of herbs or soil needed for planting and tending to the garden. A microscope is also a must-have for diagnostically identifying any pests, diseases, or contaminants within your garden. Using stirring rods, you can properly mix fertilizers to provide lasting nutrition to your herbs, while test tubes and beakers let you measure out hydroponic nutrients with ecological efficiency. With laboratory tools in hand, even first-time gardeners can develop an abundance of beautiful herbs and plants.

Tips and Tricks to Consider

For a successful herb garden, it's vital to consider factors such as light, water, and soil. But there's more to it than that. Here are a few tips and tricks to bear in mind when creating an herb garden:

A. Companion Planting

An essential component of a successful herb garden is companion planting. Combining herbs with vegetables and flowers in your garden can introduce beneficial insects, improve soil quality, and protect plants from pests. Cultivating herbs close to other crops may increase their potential yield as well. For example, pairing tomato plants with basil will not only block weeds but also improves the flavor of both crops. Consider planting tall herbs like dill or fennel near a trellis for climbing beans and peas. This will offer more surface area for the climbing vines while providing shade from the sun's rays. Additionally, planting chives next to roses naturally wards off pests without introducing harsh chemicals. Utilizing companion planting techniques in your herb garden will ensure healthy growth and the tastiest possible harvests!

B. Soil Amendments

Enhancing your herb garden with soil amendments is a great way to get the most out of your plants. Not only can you create nutrient-rich soil that helps the herbs thrive, but using organic amendments also helps the environment in the long run. Compost tea, manure, and mulch are great additions and will provide a delicate balance of minerals and nutrients for optimal growth. Additionally, adding perlite or vermiculite will help aerate the soil, improving water retention while also creating a more structured base. This simple maintenance tip can create an enhanced atmosphere for your herbs!

C. Growing Herbs Indoors

Discover the delight of having fresh herbs on hand all year long by cultivating them indoors. Not only do they season and enhance almost any dish, but the aromas of many common herbs can also lift your mood and create a pleasant atmosphere in the home. To get the most from your indoor herb garden, ensure you're picking out plants that are suitable for an indoor ecosystem. Some herbs require lots of sunlight, making them better suited for outdoor gardening. You also need to ensure that you're fertilizing at least once every two weeks because herbs can deplete a lot of soil nutrients quickly. Finally, if you want to step up your game, many herbs like basil will thrive when placed near windows in a DIY hydroponic setup.

D. Vertical Gardening

Vertical gardening brings new life to traditional herb gardens with its unique design and space-saving features. This alternative form of gardening allows you to make the best use of your outdoor living areas while providing plenty of room for your herbs to thrive and flourish. Give your plants plenty of sunlight and nutrition by utilizing vertical growing systems such as shelves, trellises, obelisks, hanging baskets, or wall planters to create a vibrant display that's also easy to maintain. Plus, it's fun and rewarding to see how plants adapt to their new environment! With vertical gardening for your herb garden, there are endless possibilities for you to discover and explore.

E. Popular Herb Varieties to Plant

Planting an herb garden is a great way to access herbal antibiotics, and a few varieties are known for their medicinal benefits. Herbs like echinacea, oregano, and rosemary can be used to ward off infections and easily be grown in most climates. The immune-boosting properties of echinacea make it great for when you're starting to feel under the weather. Oregano has antibacterial qualities to prevent bacterial illness and is used as an ingredient in sauces and marinades. Finally, rosemary can help fight away fungi while adding fragrance and flavor to many dishes. It's also delicious when roasted with potatoes!

F. Additional Tips and Tricks

When it comes to herb gardening, there are a few additional tips and tricks to keep in mind. First, pick a location that is full of sunshine, has good air circulation, and preferably is close to a water source. An outdoor herb garden will generally need six hours of direct sunlight per day, while an indoor one needs eight or more. In addition, the soil should be well-drained and cultivated with lots of compost. Herbs prefer soils rich in organic matter, so make sure to add lots of compost or aged manure. Preparing the soil is also essential for a successful herb garden. Try to use light and airy soil, such as those found in sandy loam or heavy clay soils. The soil should be tilled or broken down to allow the roots plenty of room to grow. It should also be fertilized with a balanced fertilizer to ensure the right nutrients are present.

An herb garden is an easy, cost-effective way to get a supply of fresh herbs right at your fingertips. You can choose which herbs you want and grow them in your own space without having to worry about purchasing expensive grocery store herbs that might be imported from far-off places. By growing it yourself, you're sure to get the freshest possible product every time. Plus, using your homegrown herbs will add a delicious flair to dishes that you wouldn't be able to achieve with store-bought herbs. An herb garden won't require too much maintenance and is a great way to save some money while still enjoying all your favorite herbs.

This chapter has focused on the basics of growing an herb garden and building an herb lab. It is crucial to select the right space, prepare the soil properly, and select the right herbs for you to get the most out of your herb garden. Growing an herb garden will allow you to have a constant supply of fresh herbs at your fingertips, plus allow you to make your herbal medicines. With the right tools, knowledge, and dedication, you can easily start your herb lab and be on your way to creating natural medicines. Remember, the key to success is in preparation, so take your time and research the best ways to get your herb garden and lab up and running! Good luck!

Chapter 5

Safety Tips and Tricks

Herbal antibiotics have grown increasingly popular in recent years for treating infections, offering an all-natural and holistic approach to well-being. While their powerful effects can be beneficial to many remedial needs, it is also crucial to understand their potential drawbacks. For instance, they may not be as potent as synthetic or pharmaceutical drugs and could therefore require longer treatment sessions with repeated dosing. In addition, natural herbal medicines can cause unexpected interactions when combined with prescribed medications, which makes it critical that those seeking out these remedies understand what they are taking and speak openly with their doctors.

With knowledge comes the potential to heal in new and healthier ways, so understanding these common concerns and limitations of herbal antibiotics will help maximize the benefits of this approach to wellness. This chapter will discuss the potential drawbacks and limitations of herbal antibiotics as well as how to ensure safety when using them. The information provided will help you make informed decisions about your health and be prepared for what to expect when taking herbal antibiotics.

Common Concerns of Herbal Antibiotics

Despite their touted health benefits, there are legitimate reasons for hesitation when using herbal antibiotics. They can cause allergic reactions due to their potential for cross-reactivity with other herbals or environmental contaminants. The dosage instructions can be unclear, so one may not get a proper therapeutic dose. Additionally, these herbal medicines do not have a standard surveillance system like conventional pharmaceuticals, so studying their composition and adverse effects is difficult. Research findings on these herbs offer highly conflicting results, making it difficult to determine if certain biological claims about them are true. For those considering herbal antibiotics, it is vital to carefully weigh all the pros and cons associated with these products before taking them.

1. Lack of FDA Approval

One of the primary concerns about herbal antibiotics is that they have not been approved by the FDA. The FDA is responsible for ensuring that medications are safe and effective before they are made available to the public. Herbal antibiotics have not undergone the same rigorous testing as conventional antibiotics, so their safety and effectiveness are not known.

2. Lack of Scientific Evidence

A major concern about herbal antibiotics is the absence of scientific proof to validate their efficacy. While some studies suggest herbal antibiotics may be effective, more research is needed to confirm these results. Additionally, it is not known if herbal antibiotics are safe for long-term use or if they can cause significant side effects.

3. Potential Drug Interactions

An additional worry regarding herbal antibiotics is their probable interference with any other medicines you are consuming. If you are taking any prescription medications, it is crucial to talk to your doctor before taking herbal antibiotics, as they could potentially interact with your other medications and cause serious side effects.

4. Quality Control Issues

Another concern about herbal antibiotics is that there may be quality control issues with products that are sold over the counter. The FDA does not regulate herbal supplements, so there is no guarantee that they contain the ingredients listed on the label or that they are safe for human consumption.

5. Cost

Another worry associated with herbal antibiotics is their potential to be pricier than the traditional antibiotic option. While some herbal antibiotics may be available over-the-counter, others may need to be purchased from a specialty retailer, which can increase the cost. Additionally, insurance companies typically do not cover the cost of herbal supplements, so you would be responsible for the entire cost yourself.

6. Allergic Reactions

Besides its efficacy, another area of concern for herbal antibiotics is potential allergic reactions in certain individuals. If you have any allergies, it is important to talk to your doctor before taking herbal antibiotics, as they could potentially trigger an allergic reaction. Symptoms of an allergic reaction include hives, swelling, difficulty breathing, and dizziness. You should seek medical attention immediately if you experience any of these symptoms after taking herbal antibiotics.

Limitations of Herbal Antibiotics

While herbal antibiotics may seem like a healthier option than traditional antibiotics, they come with their own set of limitations. Let's take a look at the strengths and weaknesses of herbal antibiotics so you can make an informed decision about whether or not they are right for you.

Strength

One limitation of herbal antibiotics is that their strength is often weaker than traditional antibiotics. This means that it may take longer to treat an infection compared to using a traditional antibiotic. Additionally, some herbal antibiotics may not be strong enough to treat serious infections, such as those caused by bacteria, fungi, or viruses. Therefore, it's crucial to speak with your doctor before using them and make sure that they are suitable for your condition.

Duration of Effectiveness

Another limitation of herbal antibiotics is their duration of effectiveness. Unlike traditional antibiotics, which typically last for several weeks or months after use, many herbal remedies only last for a few days or weeks before their effects begin to fade away. If you need long-term treatment for an infection, herbal remedies may not be the best choice.

Accessibility

A third limitation of herbal antibiotics is their accessibility. Many herbs used in these remedies can only be found in certain parts of the world and may not be widely available in other regions or countries. Additionally, some herbs used in these remedies can only be obtained through special orders from online retailers or health food stores, making them difficult to obtain if you don't live near one of these establishments.

Expense

Herbal antibiotics also tend to be more expensive than traditional medications due to the cost associated with obtaining rare herbs from around the world as well as the cost associated with producing high-quality products containing these herbs. Therefore, if cost is an issue, then investing in high-quality herbal remedies may not be financially feasible for everyone depending on their financial situation and budgeting needs.

Reliability

Finally, there are also some questions about the reliability and efficacy of many herbal antibiotic treatments due to limited scientific research on this topic and lack of consistency between different brands or manufacturers when it comes to dosing instructions and ingredient lists, which can make it difficult to know what exactly you are getting when purchasing these products online or in stores.

While there are certainly benefits associated with utilizing natural remedies such as herbal antibiotics over traditional medications, there are also some limitations that must be considered before deciding whether or not this type of treatment is right for you. Make sure you speak with your doctor about any potential risks and side effects associated with using these types of treatments before making any decisions so that you can make an informed choice about what will work best for your individual needs and circumstances.

Ensuring Safety When Using Herbal Antibiotics

It is crucial to take a few precautions when using natural remedies to ensure your safety and maximize the efficacy of the treatment. Here are 5 tips for using herbal antibiotics safely:

1. Researching Herbs

Before taking any herbal remedy, research the herbs you plan on using. Some herbs will be more beneficial than others, depending on what you are trying to treat. It is also crucial to understand the potential side effects associated with each herb so that you can make an informed decision about which one is best suited for your needs.

2. Quality of Ingredients

Quality matters when it comes to herbal antibiotics, so use high-quality ingredients in your remedies. Make sure that the herbs and other ingredients you use are organic and free from pesticides or other chemicals that can interfere with their effectiveness. Some companies offer pre-made herbal remedies free from toxins, so this may be a good option if you don't want to buy all the individual ingredients yourself.

3. Evaluating Allergies

Certain herbs may cause allergic reactions in some people, so evaluate any allergies before taking herbal antibiotics. Even if a certain herb is generally safe, there may be a risk of developing an allergy if you are sensitive to certain plant compounds or pollens. If possible, try testing out small amounts of each herb before committing to a full course of treatment.

4. Consulting with a Professional

Before embarking on any form of self-treatment, it's always best practice to consult with a healthcare professional first. This ensures that any illnesses or conditions are properly diagnosed and treated with an appropriate plan tailored specifically for you. A qualified healthcare practitioner can also recommend specific herbs or combinations of herbs that will be most effective for your condition based on their knowledge and experience with herbal medicines.

5. Monitoring Side Effects

As with all treatments, monitor side effects while taking herbal antibiotics and seek medical help if necessary. Common side effects include nausea, dizziness, headaches, skin rashes or irritations, upset stomach, diarrhea, and constipation. Keeping track of how you feel during treatment can help identify any issues quickly so that medical professionals can address them appropriately if needed.

What to Expect When Using Herbal Antibiotics

Herbal antibiotics contain various healing herbs, vitamins, and minerals, so depending on the specific product that is used, the effects can vary. For example, certain products may cause certain symptoms like diarrhea or an upset stomach which could potentially be reduced when taken with food. Additionally, they can take anywhere from several weeks to several months to fully take effect in treating minor bacterial infections. All in all, understanding what to expect when taking herbal antibiotics is critical for the best results and overall safety.

Immediate Relief

Herbal antibiotics can provide much-needed relief from the discomfort of minor illnesses. Although it's essential to address any symptoms dealt with professional medical attention, for common complaints, herbal antibiotics are a safe alternative. They offer natural remedies that can be taken without having to worry about side effects and antibiotic resistance. Generally, you can expect to start feeling the benefits in 24 hours, but usually, it takes closer to a week for full results.

Herbal antibiotics can provide almost instant relief from symptoms such as fever, inflammation, and pain due to their anti-inflammatory properties. Some herbs used in herbal antibiotic preparations are effective against certain types of bacteria that cause infection. For example, garlic is effective against Escherichia coli (E.coli), which causes urinary tract infections or salmonella poisoning.

Treatment will involve taking tablets, suspensions, or tinctures for up to two months. Clear instructions are normally provided with each order, and these instructions must be followed closely to get the most out of your herbal treatments. Over time, you should begin to notice your body responding positively, and the effectiveness of herbal antibiotics is often hard to argue with.

Long-Term Effects

The long-term effects of using herbal antibiotics are worth considering when assessing your health care needs. When used for prolonged periods, these natural remedies can improve your immune system and enhance the overall function of your body's various systems. Because each herb has its own set of benefits, you should consult with a certified healthcare provider to discuss which one is best for your particular situation before beginning a course of treatment.

Herbal antibiotics can provide relief from infectious illness, inflammation, and chronic pain. However, if not taken as directed, there may be potential risks such as allergic reactions or unwanted side effects. Remember that herbal medicines do not count as true medical treatments, and it's best to use them in tandem with whatever conventional care you may already be receiving from your doctor or healthcare practitioner.

Possible Risks

Herbal antibiotics offer an alternative to conventional prescription antibiotics, but potential risks remain. It's essential to be aware of the potential issues associated with herbal antibacterial, such as the lack of scientific studies on the benefits and risks associated with these treatments. While many believe that herbal remedies can treat illnesses, no empirical evidence forms the basis of these claims.

Additionally, certain herbs can cause side effects such as upset stomachs, nausea, headaches, dizziness, and sedation. Users may also experience adverse reactions when using herbal antibiotics with other drugs. It is advisable to consult a medical professional before attempting any form of self-medication or treatment. Even though natural remedies can provide relief from mild infections and ailments without serious side effects, caution should be used when investigating their use in treating more serious illnesses.

Safety Tips When Using Herbal Antibiotics

Herbal antibiotics are becoming more popular and can effectively fight infection, but safety should always be a priority. The most crucial step is to ensure that the herbs you purchase for a homemade remedy are of the highest quality and sourced from reliable and trusted vendors. Before rushing into treating yourself with herbal antibiotics, consult your doctor or health practitioner about any potential interactions, as some herbs may interact with medications.

Some herbs require extra preparation before being taken, so research them carefully and make sure to follow directions properly. With the following safety tips in mind, herbal antibiotics can be a powerful tool in your natural healing arsenal.

1. Take the Correct Dosage

When taking herbal antibiotics, remember to always follow the recommended dosage. Taking too much of an herbal antibiotic can cause the same problems that taking too much of a conventional antibiotic can, such as upset stomach, vomiting, and diarrhea. Taking too little may not be effective for treating an illness or infection either. Be sure to read all instructions when using any type of medication. Herbal antibiotics have many benefits, and taking them in the correct dosage is essential for experiencing their full effects and safety.

2. Store Herbs Properly

It is vital to store herbs properly to maintain their medicinal properties. Herbs should be stored in a cool, dark place away from any sources of moisture, such as sinks, showers, and windowsills. They should also be kept away from areas such as stoves and ovens that may produce heat or steam. Label your herbs to get the full benefit of the herb without accidentally mixing up different components. If stored correctly, these natural remedies can provide great healing properties without the worry of any dangerous side effects.

3. Avoid Using if You Have Allergies

Herbal antibiotics, while considered natural medicine and often perceived as being safe and free of side effects, can act as antihistamines, the same commonly prescribed medications used to treat allergies. However, because governmental bodies do not regulate them, people unknowingly risk experiencing irritating skin rashes as an allergic reaction. Be aware of this possibility when choosing to use herbal antibiotics, as certain ingredients may set off reactions in individuals prone to allergies.

While they may offer a more natural approach to healing, being informed will save its users a lot of discomfort. Those who suffer from allergies should take extra caution and use these treatments with a knowledgeable medical professional. A qualified doctor can advise on dosage and ingredients to ensure that patients are safely able to go forward with their treatment plan. If you have allergies, err on the side of caution and speak with your physician before beginning any herbal antibiotic regimen.

4. Discontinue Use if Symptoms Worsen

Be aware of any changing symptom patterns while taking herbal antibiotics, as these could be indicative of an adverse reaction. If worse symptoms begin to show during treatment, you should discontinue use right away and consult a medical professional. An uncontrolled reaction could lead to an increase in severity or even serious health complications. Be sure to stay vigilant while supplementing your routine with herbal antibiotics to ensure that they are used safely and correctly. Discontinuing use if your symptoms worsen is a safety precaution when using herbal antibiotics to ensure that your health is carefully monitored for any unforeseen issues.

5. Allow Time for Herbal Antibiotics to Work

When using herbal antibiotics to treat an illness, it is necessary to allow adequate time for them to work. Herbal antibiotics are often slower-acting than conventional antibacterial drugs, so practitioners recommend giving herbs plenty of time to take effect to maximize their healing potential. This can be difficult when feeling better is the desired outcome, but patience is essential if you wish to avoid risking a relapse. The key is learning how long each supplement should be taken before deciding on whether or not it's working and looking into alternative remedies if need be. Keep in mind that consistency when taking the right herbal supplements will result in stronger immunity and better overall health in the long run.

6. Keep Track of Your Progress

Taking herbal antibiotics can be incredibly helpful when it comes to improving your health and well-being, but it is crucial to track your progress. Monitoring your health throughout taking herbal antibiotics can give you useful insights into the benefits they have on your body. It's always a good idea to keep a journal and make a note of changes in the amount of energy or mental clarity you experience. Additionally, be sure to pay attention to any other changes, such as new symptoms or improved functioning, and document them to feel confident about taking these powerful herbs with safety in mind.

Herbal antibiotics offer a natural alternative to many harsh and powerful prescription medications, which can sometimes have some pretty unpleasant side effects. Knowing the best and safest way to use any type of herbal antibiotic is crucial to ensuring that you get maximum relief while minimizing the risk of any adverse reactions. While herbal antibiotics may be sold in many health food and online stores without a doctor's recommendation, consulting with an expert, such as a certified nutritionist or medical herbalist, for information about the appropriate dose and recommended length of time for taking an herbal remedy, is essential for preventing potential dangers.

Additionally, just because something is called "natural" does not mean it comes without potential drawbacks. Always read labels carefully and make sure that you understand what all of the ingredients are before consuming anything. With these guidelines in mind, it's possible to enjoy the benefits of herbal antibiotics without sacrificing your health.

Chapter 6

Tips and Tricks for
Harvesting and Preparing

To have the most effective results from naturally occurring herbal antibiotics, selecting and harvesting herbs in peak condition is crucial. Failure to pay attention to harvesting times and the maturity of each herb can result in less potent medicine and a much greater risk of ineffective or even hazardous concoctions. The quality of herbs used for herbal antibiotics depends on understanding when each herb should be harvested for maximum medicinal value.

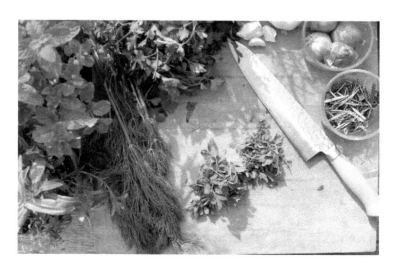

Experienced herbalists can tell whether an herb has reached its essential peak just by inspecting its scent, texture, color, and size. Many traditional cultures around the world have been using herbs to fight infection and sickness for centuries through their knowledge of harvesting the right parts at exactly the right time. When done correctly, this process helps ensure the strongest medicinal power out of every single herb included in an antibacterial tincture or syrup.

This chapter will provide an overview of all the steps involved in gathering and harvesting herbs, from selecting the best specimens to using proper cutting or handpicking techniques. It will also cover the most important herb parts used to create herbal antibiotics and preventive measures to avoid plant damage. This guide aims to help herbalists and other interested parties gain a deeper understanding of proper harvesting techniques that will lead to more potent medicine.

Herb Parts Used in Herbal Antibiotics

Different parts of herbs may be used to effectively create herbal antibiotics, such as root extractions or essential oils. In some cases, the potency of herbal antibiotics can be enhanced by combining multiple herbs into a single formula. Herbal antibiotics should always be used in combination with other healthcare protocols. By doing so, we can benefit from the broad spectrum activity of herbal defenses while also building our own body's natural immunity and vitality.

1. Roots

The healing properties used in many herbs contribute to the popularity of herbal antibiotics. In particular, certain roots like turmeric, neem, ginger, and garlic are effective in treating bacterial infections due to their antibacterial, antifungal, and antiviral compounds. Roots are part of many herbal remedies and can even be made into syrups or ointments for better absorption into the body. By researching some of the more popular roots used in herbal antibiotics, people can start making more informed decisions about their healthcare needs.

2. Leaves

Leaves are used in many herbal medicines and natural home remedies for their antibiotic properties. Herbal antibiotics made using leaves can be used to treat a variety of bacterial infections and other illnesses, such as viruses and fungi. As effective treatments, these remedies have been around for centuries, certainly before the discovery of synthetic antibiotics. Leaf-based herbal antibiotics are readily available from health food stores, online sources, and many local apothecaries. These remedies can be ingested as teas or tinctures or applied directly to the affected area as ointments or poultices. While herbal antibiotics may not always be as potent as pharmaceuticals, they are an effective natural alternative that can help to treat minor illnesses more gently than harsher drugs.

3. Stems

Stems are the major structural supports of plants, yet they are also used for medicinal purposes. Herbal antibiotics rely on certain parts of stems to help conquer bacterial infections. Extracts from coneflower, Chinese skullcap, and Echinacea stem bark have all been shown to be significantly effective in inhibiting the growth and spread of bacteria. Furthermore, many plants stem compounds also possess antibacterial properties against antibiotic-resistant pathogens like MRSA. Stems can thus be a powerful herbal remedy for treating common ailments, as long as they are responsibly gathered concerning the environment and ecological structure.

4. Flowers

Flowers are an integral part of many herbal antibiotic preparations, with various parts of flowers helping to promote health and wellness. For example, herbs such as calendula, chamomile, and echinacea often rely on the flower to provide many beneficial compounds. In particular, the petals of these flowers have been identified as one of the most efficient components in promoting healthy immunity. While each flower may vary in color and size, its medicinal effects remain constant, providing our bodies with vital minerals and allowing us to make use of essential antioxidants. Along with diets rich in fruits and vegetables for a balanced lifestyle, incorporating flowers into our healthcare routine can give us that extra boost toward well-being.

5. Seeds

From its rich oils and nourishing nutrients, the herbaceous portion of seeds can be used to create a powerful herbal antibiotic. They are often known for their antiviral, antibacterial, antifungal, and other medicinal powers. Some have antioxidant abilities to assist with cellular health. Herbal antibiotics may not work for everyone, but those who experiment with and find success with plant-based remedies have a powerful tool at their disposal for fighting infection. By harnessing the natural properties of herbs, smart practitioners can craft remedies that quite literally sow new life in a struggling body.

Proper Harvesting of Herb Parts

To ensure the highest quality and greatest yield, it is vital to familiarize yourself with how to harvest herbs properly. Neglecting to pick at the right time or in an appropriate manner could lead to disappointing results. The season, stage of growth, and type of herb should all be taken into consideration when making a plan for harvesting. Some herbs benefit from being cut before full maturity, while others require them to reach their peak before they're gathered. In either case, the proper techniques must be used during harvesting practices. Knowing how to assess when the right time comes and utilizing techniques to properly collect herbs without damaging them is a key part of cultivating an optimal yield.

1. Selecting the Best Time of the Year

When it comes to harvesting the parts of herbs, timing is critical. Every herb has its own 'harvest window,' a point in time when components of the plant reach their peak nutritive value and flavor. When these windows pass, the plant begins to wilt or go through developments that render it unremarkable. Therefore, selecting the best time to harvest is crucial for anyone looking to enjoy peak flavors and nutrition from their herbs. While some parts of specific plants are better harvested at different moments in their growth cycle, many will provide top-quality results around mid-summer as long as certain precautions are taken. The key is making sure to do your research beforehand regarding which parts should be harvested and when to ensure you get the freshest and most flavorful produce out of your efforts!

2. Quantity to Harvest

Harvesting herbs at the right time and stage of the herb's cycle can ensure their flavored essential oils are at their peak. To obtain the best flavor, select herbs to harvest early in the morning, after the dew has evaporated, but before the hot sun dissipates oils that give plants their flavor. The amount of herb parts to harvest also depends on when you plan to use them. For example, if you plan to dry your leaves for future use, cut more than if you're harvesting for immediate use. Fresh herbs can be pinched off with your fingers or snipped off with scissors and should come from the ends of branches rather than cutting back entire stems each time and allowing for regrowth before mining the plant again.

3. Cut, Don't Pull

When it's time to collect the parts of herbs, you can choose whether to cut or pull. In many cases, cutting is the preferred method. This reduces the chances of harming your plant and allows for more control above the desired output. These cuts must be precise and measured. To ensure only the parts meant to be harvested are collected, begin snipping from the top down when harvesting individual herb sprigs and cut stems at an angle so that some leaf nodes on both sides remain intact. If cutting too far back from the desired point, wait until there is enough growth before harvesting again, as this will allow for quick regeneration of what was lost. With proper technique, enjoy a healthy harvest of useful plant parts for all your culinary needs!

4. Leave Enough for Regeneration

Herbs are a wonderful addition to any garden, adding vibrant color, flavor, aroma, and even medicinal benefits. But if you're looking to maximize the value of your herb garden, it's crucial to properly harvest your herbs. When harvesting herbs, it leaves leaves and stems behind so the plant can regenerate. Otherwise, you won't be able to enjoy your herbs over a long period as they will die out quickly due to lack of nutrition and water when too much is taken away.

Most herb leaves should be harvested in the morning before the heat of the day sets in, and most flower buds should be harvested at their peak, but if possible, try leaving some flowers behind so that more come up next season. Harvesting herbs help stimulate growth and encourages business, resulting in greater yields in upcoming harvests. To ensure an abundant harvest of herbs over an extended period, practice proper harvesting techniques such as scavenging from each plant rather than stripping or cutting all of one variety from one plant at once.

5. Properly Dry and Store Herbs

Herbs have been used for centuries in many different dishes, medicinal treatments, and more. To ensure the best quality and taste of those herbs, it is crucial to properly dry and store them. Harvesting the right parts of the herb is a large part of ensuring top-notch flavor and freshness. Knowing which edible parts of the herb will help a person determine when it's time to harvest and what parts need to be taken off before drying or storing.

Leaves should be harvested when relatively young for maximum flavor. Some herbs, such as basil and oregano, need to be picked before they flower, while others should be harvested after they flower. Seeds should be collected just before being released by the plant. Roots require patience. They don't become edible until bulbous or fibrous enough for human consumption, and their tastes vary depending on the type of herb collected. While it can take practice, understanding proper harvesting techniques can make a big difference in preparing your herbal remedies.

Cutting or Picking Techniques and Tools

To ensure the maximum flavor and quality of herbs, handling them properly when harvesting is essential. Knowing the right cutting or picking techniques and tools to use can help in this process. Herbs can be harvested with garden scissors, pruning shears, or by pinching and plucking with your hands. Selective harvest with shortcuts preserves herb leaves best and prevents damage to stems. Pruning back herbs will promote bushier growth and encourage more foliage production overall. When harvesting whole branches or stems, it is best to grab them just under where they connect to the larger plant structure and pull away in one motion, which ensures a clean break. A sharp pair of scissors works well for neatly tying off at the top of cuttings for easy transporting for drying if desired. These tips will ensure your herbs are handled with care for optimal harvesting results!

1. Handpicking

Proper harvesting of herb parts is essential to ensure a quality crop, and one way to do this is through handpicking. Though there are machines available, manual labor is the more cost-effective approach that consistently gives the best results. A successful handpicking process requires individuals with an intricate knowledge of the varied characteristics of each herb and a keen eye for detail. Depending on the type of plant and its intended outcome, handpicked must gather either its leaves or buds, identifying potential pests and discarding any wilted or unacceptable specimens. Those with an eye for detail will have no difficulty successfully harvesting fully ripe herbal parts, ensuring top-notch products for customers' satisfaction.

2. Snipping

Harvesting herbs for health remedies can be a fulfilling task. Different herb parts may need to be harvested at different times, but timely and methodical snipping is key to the proper growth of the plant. Once you decide which herb parts will best suit your needs, examine the plant closely and make small intentional cuts above a leaf node, leaving a few pairs of leaves on the stem to encourage further growth. Being mindful of when and how much to take ensures that there will still be plenty of renewable stock and ensures future harvests all season long!

3. Using Tools

Using the right tools is an essential step in the proper harvesting of herb parts. Pruning shears or scissors are best to use since they provide a clean cut and avoid bruising or tearing of the leaves, which can reduce the quality of the herbs. For weeds with shallow roots, ensure that the entire root system has been pulled out while harvesting them. A garden trowel or Hori Hori knife may come in handy to get at tougher roots. Strong gloves should be worn when handling these tools as well as when pulling weeds from the ground to protect hands from harm. Taking great care and having the proper tools ensures that you can enjoy your freshly harvested herbs at their fullest potential with robust taste and aroma!

Damage Prevention Techniques

To achieve an optimal yield of herbal plants, it is essential to employ proper harvesting techniques when gathering the herbs' parts. Before harvesting, the best time and place should be considered since weather conditions, and light exposure can affect the volume of active compounds in the plant. After deciding where to harvest, take care to only pluck one layer at a time, starting from the outside of the herb and working inward. This will ensure that there will still be enough growth for another harvest later on. Finally, since dried herbs are more potent than fresh ones due to loss of moisture content, store them away from sunlight in airtight containers once harvesting is complete. Following these steps can effectively prevent damage while getting the most out of any herb-based project.

1. Leave Some Leaves

While it's common for plants to suffer from damage due to a variety of factors, such as harsh weather, keenly observe and assess any damage done before harvesting. This is especially crucial if utilizing parts of the herb for medicinal uses. Often, leaving some of the leaves on damaged plants can give them a better chance of recovering and becoming healthy again. So don't forget that not all the leaves need to be trimmed. After all, providing healthy plants with proper care will result in bountiful harvests while reducing wastage.

2. Don't Overwater

Growing herbs is one of the most rewarding experiences for gardeners, but over-watering is one of the most common mistakes. As this can damage the plants, it's critical to remember that a consistent watering schedule is essential for growing healthy herbs. Overwatering can lead to root rot, which can kill entire plants, impeding your ability to harvest useful herbs like basil and oregano. Taking steps to avoid overwatering and dealing quickly with any damaged plants are critically important in getting a successful harvest from your herb garden. Setting up a simple drip system or other timed irrigation can help make sure your precious herbs are appropriately watered at just the right time and intensity.

3. Maintain Healthy Soil

Maintaining healthy soil is essential for harvesting herb parts properly. Gardening should be a long-term process and should not be overdone in terms of time and energy investment. If you take the time to nourish your soil with organic matter, such as compost or aged manure, it will reward you with rich rewards for years to come. Along with quality soil nutrition, water also plays an essential role in healthy plant growth. By watering at different times of the day and adding more water, when necessary, you can keep your soil from becoming dry and enable your plants to reach their full potential. Finally, you can use mulch above ground to help conserve moisture below ground and prevent weeds from getting the better of your crop.

Dealing with Damaged Plants

Proper harvesting of herb parts is essential for maintaining healthy plants and producing high-quality yields. Knowing when to harvest and how to appropriately collect herb parts can be the difference between damaged plants and thriving ones. First, inspect your plants for signs of disease, wilting, or lack of overall health. If these issues are present, it may be best to wait or look into options such as pruning or flowering before harvesting a plant's parts.

Next, proper cutting techniques should be followed when collecting parts like flowers and leaves; the most effective way is to pick the right above-ground portions without reaching too far down to avoid damaging the roots. Also, try cutting only what you need at that moment. Storage tends to decrease herb part quality over time, so opting for short-term solutions like saving seeds from certain herbs can prove invaluable in the future.

1. Isolate the Plant

Isolating damaged plants from the rest of the garden is essential in ensuring that only healthy herb parts are harvested for consumption.

This practice can help keep diseases, pests, and weeds from spreading throughout the entire garden by isolating any infected areas before more problems arise. Using mulch sheets, thick shears, or rubber gloves to manipulate plant parts instead of manually touching them can also help prevent additional damage and cross-contamination from person to person.

2. Monitor for Pests

Keeping plants healthy and free of pests is essential to proper harvesting. When pests have damaged the herbs you're growing, it can take longer to harvest correctly and yield smaller results. The best way to ensure healthy herb plants is to regularly inspect and monitor for pests, as catching any infestations early can help reduce damage. Look for chewed leaves or stems, spots, sickly yellow or brown patches, or spunky webbings that indicate insect activity. If caught soon enough, taking preventive measures like hand-picking bugs off your plants can work wonders, while severe cases may require stronger methods such as applying chemical treatments.

3. Give the Plant Time to Recover

While patience is key when dealing with harvesting and caring for herbs, it is especially critical if your herb plants are particularly damaged. Assess the plant and use various techniques, such as trimming off any dead leaves to help prevent further damage or disrepair, rotating containers around a light source to promote even growth, and providing adequate nutrition for recovery. Taking the time for healing before harvest will give the herbs the best chance at successful regrowth and future harvests. Make sure you wait until visible signs of improvement occur before attempting to harvest parts of the plant again.

Harvesting herbs can be a tricky process, but with the right steps, you can ensure that your herb plants remain healthy and productive. Properly assessing a plant before harvest, monitoring for pests, isolating any damaged plants, and giving the herb time to heal all play an important role in the successful harvesting of herbs. With these helpful tips, you'll be more confident in your herb-harvesting abilities and better prepared to provide your garden with the best herbs it can produce.

Chapter 7

Herbal Medicine Making Handbook

Herbal medicine is a form of therapy that is growing in popularity. It is an effective and natural way of healing and improving physical, mental, and emotional health. Herbal medicine has been used for centuries in many cultures and is still used today to treat a variety of ailments in people all over the world. Different forms of herbal medicine have different benefits, and each has its unique advantages.

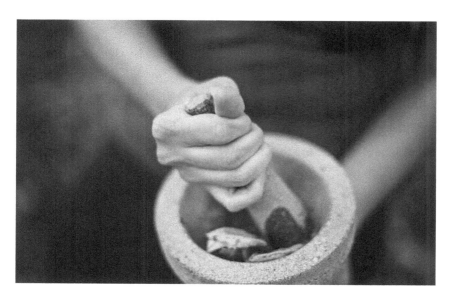

The tools needed to make herbal medicine are simple, and the process is easy. Furthermore, growing your herbs has many benefits. This chapter will explain everything related to making medicine using herbs. Different forms of herbal medicine, the tools needed, and the importance of having a herb garden to make medicine will also be discussed. By the end of this chapter, you should have a better understanding of how to make herbal medicine from home.

Different Forms of Herbal Medicine

It is essential to understand the various herbal remedies available when looking for a natural healing option. Each has its unique benefits, so weigh your options carefully and decide what treatment is best for you. While traditional Chinese herbal medicine typically involves a mixture of ground-up herbs and pieces of root, Ayurvedic Herbal Medicine utilizes more individualized treatments based on a person's balance between energy levels.

Throughout Europe, the practice looks different yet again with the presence of single-herb sprays, creams, teas, powders, syrups, and ointments. And for those looking for something a bit unusual or original to try out, there are other forms like Biography's Personal Health Mapping or Doscher's Live Cell Therapy. Regardless of what type you are drawn to, there's always something that can provide relief from doctor-prescribed drugs without sacrificing effectiveness or quality.

1. Decoctions

Decoctions are one of the oldest forms of herbal medicine and have been used for centuries in cultures around the world. They involve boiling herbs to extract their beneficial properties, then letting them cool and drinking them as tea. Decoctions can be an effective way to quickly get vitamins and minerals from herbal sources into the body, supporting overall health and well-being.

Herbalists often recommend taking decoctions regularly to maintain wellness, or they may suggest them specifically for ailments such as common colds. Decoctions offer an easy way to add natural remedies to your diet without having to shop around for hard-to-find ingredients or take complicated mixtures of pills or liquid supplements. Taking a decoction can be as simple as boiling water with a handful of herbs that you already have on hand. It is a great way to experience the power of nature with minimal effort!

2. Infusions

One type of herbal medicine that is surging in popularity is infusions. An infusion combines the best of traditional medicines, like teas and tisanes, with therapeutic benefits from herbs. These infusions are made from liquid extracts of flowers, leaves, bark, roots, and even fruit. With different combinations available, infusions offer a tailor-made approach to herbal health for everyone. Through proper guidance and research into their one-of-a-kind recipes, individuals can take advantage of the therapeutic benefits that various herbs have to offer with unique drinks perfect for any palate. For those looking to gain access to many different forms of herbal medicine with ease, there's no better option than investing in high-quality herbal infusions.

3. Teas

Tea has been used as an herbal medicine for centuries by many cultures across the globe. The use of tea dates back to 2737 B.C. when Chinese Emperor Shen Nung is credited with first introducing this popular beverage. There are different forms of teas, each providing unique health benefits that have been studied and documented throughout history. Green tea, white tea, oolong tea, black tea, and Pu-erh tea all come from the Camellia sinensis plant species, while herbal teas are based on flowers, stems, roots, and other plants from a variety of sources. Drinking these different forms of tea can be a great way to easily supplement your diet in ways that serve both to nourish your body and energize your mind.

4. Tinctures

Tinctures are one of the most popular forms of herbal medicine, often seen as a natural alternative to pharmaceuticals. These liquid extracts are made by steeping an herb in a solution of alcohol, vinegar, or glycerin for weeks at a time. By doing this, it extracts the powerful components from the plant that contains medicinal properties. Once extracted, tinctures can then be dropped under the tongue or added to food or drinks for easier ingestion.

Along with being a potent and long-lasting form of medicine, tinctures are also convenient and easy to transport. There is something special about making tinctures yourself; collecting the herbs, steeping them, and feeling the power of healing through traditional methods centuries ago people have still used today. As more people become aware of this type of herbal medicine, they can look forward to exploring new ways to use tinctures since there is a wide range available!

5. Poultices

Poultices have been a form of herbal medicine that has been in existence since ancient times. Strips of wet cloth are applied directly on the skin to deliver the healing powers of specific herbs. In today's world, poultices remain a popular choice for treating various maladies, ranging from joint pain to insect bites. These treatments are incredibly versatile as they can be made with fresh or dried herbs and applied for short or extended lengths of time.

Recent evidence suggests that poultices may even be effective at relieving the pain associated with some more serious conditions, such as rheumatoid arthritis. Whether you make your herbal poultices at home or buy specialized products from a health store, it's becoming increasingly clear that this ancient form of medicine still has a lot to offer modern society.

6. Ointments

Ointments are semi-solid preparation made from herbs, wax, and fat that is applied topically to the skin. Popular examples include calendula ointment for wound healing, chamomile ointment for its anti-inflammatory properties, St John's wort ointment for bruises and painful muscles, and eucalyptus ointment for colds and respiratory ailments. Each type has its healing abilities, making them an excellent alternative to over-the-counter medications. These different forms of herbal medicine can effectively treat common issues without the harsh side effects associated with many traditional treatments.

7. Syrups

With the rise of natural health remedies, many people are now turning to syrups as a form of herbal medicine. Syrups offer many advantages over other remedies and can be used in a variety of different ways. They are easier to take than pills and are often less expensive than over-the-counter medications. Additionally, syrups, by definition, do not contain alcohol, so they provide more immediate relief without worrying about the possible effects of alcohol on your body. On top of that, syrups may often have fewer side effects due to containing lower concentrations of active ingredients than other forms of medicines. From people with diabetes looking to regulate their blood sugar levels naturally to people with allergies seeking relief from persistent cold symptoms, syrups are becoming increasingly popular as an all-natural remedy for various ailments.

8. Salves

A salve consists of natural ingredients, like herbs and essential oils, bound together with wax or oil. From ancient Egyptians to Native Americans, people around the world have used salves to soothe broken skin and heal wounds due to their anti-inflammatory properties. People today still commonly make use of herbal salves for issues such as eczema, acne, inflammation, and even insect bites. Making your herbal salve at home is incredibly easy and allows you to tailor the ingredients to your specific needs. With just a few supplies from your local health store and some patience, you can whip up a unique healing balm that is sure to improve the well-being of yourself or someone else.

Tools Needed for Making Medicine with Herbs

Making medicine from herbs requires a few special tools. While some of these implements can be found around the home, such as a mortar and pestle for grinding, others may need to be acquired from an apothecary or online supplier. A knife or herb-stripping tool is essential for removing leaves and flowers from stems. Spatulas help in transferring mixtures into containers safely. Droppers are also useful for dispensing measured amounts of tinctures and syrups. Cheesecloth and wooden strainers are ideal for filtering ingredients and making infusion broths. All the ingredients, equipment, and processes involved require patience, practice, and knowledge, especially when attempting to make healing medicines with herbs.

1. Mortar and Pestle

Crafting traditional medicines through the utilization of herbs is an age-old practice, and mortar and pestle are essential elements for this activity. The mortar is a bowl made of stone, wood, or metal that is used to grind pieces of herb into smaller pieces. A pestle is a tool used to crush the herbs and mix them, allowing the individual molecules of the herb to break down as it's ground up. Having access to these tools is critical for drawing out all of the medicinal benefits from the plant material. With this traditional technique, anyone can create herbal remedies from local plants, perfect for backyard gardeners or apothecary aficionados who want to get crafty in the kitchen!

2. Herbal Steamer

Herbal steamers are an effective way to make medicine with herbs and revive the holistic healing traditions of many cultures. To use a herbal steamer, one needs several tools and ingredients that are easily found. These include a heat source, empty glass jars, containers, fresh or dried herbs, cheesecloth or another type of strainer, and some type of pedestal for the container to rest on top of an anchoring material to secure it in place (such as stones). With all these tools gathered together and a patient but observant eye, you will soon be making your own medicinal herbal steam treatments!

3. Cheesecloth

Making medicine is not as simple as throwing a handful of plants into a pot. To get the most out of your herbs when creating medicine, cheesecloth is an essential ingredient for crafting effective remedies. With the right technique and careful use of cheesecloth, you can appropriately strain and separate herbal concoctions, making sure that your medicines are tailored to match your individual needs. Whether selling remedies at the market or whipping up something special for yourself, cheesecloth will ensure you get every last drop of goodness from your herbs.

4. Scissors

When embarking upon a journey to medicinal herb mastery, scissors are an essential tool that must not be overlooked. Scissors provide precision when harvesting herbs and cutting them into the appropriate-sized pieces to be turned into medicine. Not only do they come in a variety of sizes and styles, allowing each herbalist to find the right size for their needs, but they also have pointed tips that help make accurate cuts quickly. While herbalists can certainly get creative with methods of breaking down herbs without scissors, they will always remain a useful tool that provides an edge over those who don't use them.

5. Mason Jars

Mason jars have long been a popular tool for making medicine with herbs. Just like generations of folks before us, we can use them to store and prepare natural remedies at home. You can create powerful remedies such as lotions, balms, and tinctures using clean glass mason jars, fresh herbs, carrier oils, and beeswax. Other tools needed when using mason jars to make medicine include sharp scissors or a knife to chop your herbs finely, wooden spoons and bowls for blending, cheesecloth or a strainer for decanting liquid, labels for organizing, measuring tools for precision, an abundance of patience as some tinctures take weeks to steep. With just these few items, you can start gathering up the blessings from nature to alleviate common ailments and keep your health in check at home.

6. Strain

Making medicine involves straining herbs to obtain their positive properties. To do this effectively, one must possess the right tools. Strainers and cheesecloth are necessary for preparing herbal infusions and decoctions as they help to easily remove plant matter from the liquid mixtures. Additionally, a mortar and pestle are essential for grinding medicinal plants as it allows for a much finer mixture compared to just using one's hands. Whatever tools are chosen to work with plant medicine, make sure they are dedicated solely to that purpose to preserve their potency. With the right items in hand, brewing herbal remedies will be an efficient and enjoyable endeavor.

7. Funnel

Crafting medicines with herbs is a unique process that involves utilizing a funnel to complete the task. The funnel allows for the efficient and precise combination of herbs, ultimately resulting in a medicine tailored to the individual's needs. To make medicine with herbal plants, one must procure several items, including a funnel, finely chopped herbs, and boiling water. To ensure maximal efficacy of the herb's intended purpose, each ingredient must be measured and blended skillfully.

By using the funnel as opposed to other tools, unwanted particles can easily be discarded while allowing easeful transfer of various medicinally-active herbs into a cup or mug to brew tea or extract extracts. The unique qualities of each herb are more likely to be preserved when you use a funnel, enabling one to gain from the many benefits available from herbal medicines.

Benefits of Growing Your Own Herbal Medicine Garden

Cultivating an herbal medicine garden can be a rewarding experience, as it provides us with the opportunity to cultivate healing plants from our backyards. Not only can we save money by avoiding expensive store-bought medications, but we are also able to develop a deeper appreciation for the power of nature's healing energies. In addition to saving money and making valuable connections with nature, growing and harvesting herbs for medicinal purposes also ensures that the remedies we use are always fresh and of superior quality. As a bonus, we can enjoy the serenity of spending time in our herbal gardens while learning more about herbaceous plant species and gaining a greater understanding of how herbal remedies can be used safely to improve our well-being.

1. Easier Access to Herbs

As the body of scientific evidence supporting the use of herbs for healing continues to grow, more and more people are turning to herbal remedies as a first line of defense against common ailments. Growing your herbal medicine garden is an excellent way to ensure easier access to medicinal herbs while providing numerous additional benefits as well. In addition to saving money on store-bought products, you can create a garden that requires little maintenance, provides fragrant beauty, and ensures you have exactly what you need when health issues arise. Plus, it's incredibly gratifying to watch your medicinal plants come alive and flourish in your very own garden!

2. Cost Efficiency

Growing your herbal medicine garden can be an extremely cost-efficient way to treat everyday ailments. With a little knowledge, these herbs can cure a variety of minor illnesses, such as colds and stomach upset. Not only will you save money on over-the-counter medicines, but you will also be satisfied knowing that what you are ingesting is natural and chemical-free. You won't have to worry about any side effects because you grew and harvested the herbs yourself. Not only is this an economical choice for treating everyday problems, but it is also a wonderful way to gain knowledge about herbal remedies and deepen your connection with nature.

3. Knowing the Source of Your Medicine

Many of us take medicines without giving a thought to the source. However, the benefits of growing your herbal medicine garden can be immeasurable. It allows for complete control over the herbs you consume in your remedies and treatments. Growing your plants enables you to monitor their quality directly and ensure they are organic and non-GMO (Genetically Modified Organisms). You have access to fresh medicinal ingredients that make all the difference in efficacy and potency. Gardening is also an enjoyable activity full of joy, toil, and rewards, engaging all the senses through aromatic aromas and vibrant colors. And perhaps most importantly, nothing can beat having medicinal ingredients available right from your fingertips.

4. Knowing the Freshness of Your Herbs

Growing your herbal medicine garden provides you the benefit of truly knowing the freshness and potency of your herbs. With store-bought herbs, you don't know how old they are or if they have been handled properly to keep them at their peak. However, with a herb garden in your backyard, you can be sure that all your medicinal herbs have been freshly gathered and used within days of harvesting.

This is important, as plants lose many of their healing properties over time. Furthermore, most plants also contain special oils that require a bit of cultivation expertise to ensure maximum therapeutic potential, for example, when and how to best harvest them for capturing these oils. All these advantages make having an herbal medicine garden very attractive for those wishing to take full knowledge and control over their health care needs.

5. Environmentally Friendly

Growing your herbal medicine garden has many benefits for the environment. Not only does it reduce energy costs associated with growing and harvesting herbs, but it also eliminates much of the packaging and transportation needs that come from purchasing store-bought herbal medicines. It's an opportunity to build a more sustainable future by growing herb plants in our backyards or balconies. In addition to the environmental benefits, homemade herbal medicines are held to higher standards than options purchased at a pharmacy. Knowing exactly what goes into each remedy gives you confidence that it is free of fillers and other artificial ingredients, which helps protect both health and the environment. Growing your herbal medicines is not only beneficial for the environment, but it's also a rewarding experience that could lead to alternative healing solutions.

Herbal medicine is a powerful and cost-effective way to treat many everyday ailments. Growing your herbal medicine garden can provide you with top-quality ingredients while also reducing costs and increasing the freshness of your medicinal herbs. Not only that, it's a great way to connect with nature and take control of your health responsibly and sustainably. Growing herbs is an enjoyable activity that can bring countless rewards in the form of health, knowledge, and a more sustainable future. The benefits of growing your herbal medicine garden are plentiful, so don't hesitate to give it a try!

Chapter 8

Herbal Antibiotics for Headaches

Herbal remedies have become increasingly popular for relieving pain due to their natural, non-invasive nature. While many medications require approval from a doctor and can cause long-term side effects, herbal remedies offer a more accessible alternative. Specifically, herbal remedies have the potential to be highly effective in treating headaches. For instance, lavender oil can be used as an aroma therapy to relieve tension headaches, while Capsicum, commonly found in cayenne pepper, is known to provide relief from migraine issues.

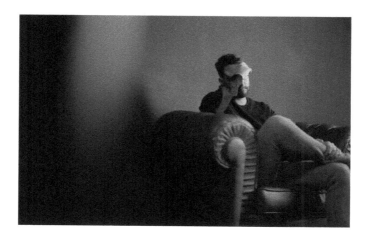

Herbal remedies are a safe and effective treatment option that may provide symptom relief with minimal risk. This chapter will explore several herbal remedies with step-by-step instructions to help you create these natural pain relief treatments at home. The ingredients and their potential benefits are listed for each recipe. With these treatments, you can relieve your headaches without resorting to costly and potentially dangerous medications.

Herbal Remedies for Headaches

From the common cold and allergies to late-night study sessions, headaches are a fact of life. Instead of turning to over-the-counter drugs and chemicals for shorter-term relief, many people have found success in herbal remedies for headaches. Herbal remedies have been used as an ancient form of healing for centuries and offer natural assistance with treating pain without any harsh side effects.

Herbs like lavender, feverfew, butterbur, and even some varieties of peppermint can be especially helpful when it comes to migraines, tension, and sinus headaches. Not only might they alleviate symptoms quickly, but they could also aid in relaxation and calming nerves. The best thing about trying out herbal remedies is that numerous home recipes help you on your way, providing tips on boiling herbs or making teas to target certain aches. Never underestimate the power of nature!

Feverfew and Valerian Tea

Many herbal treatments are available for headaches, with feverfew and valerian tea often coming up as top choices. Feverfew is a wild plant related to daisies and chamomiles that contains compounds that can help stop certain cytokines, which may be linked to migraine pain. Valerian tea has also been used for centuries in calming teas known to help reduce stress, which can be a contributing factor to headaches. Drinking the tea steeped from either of these herbs can offer not only medicinal benefits but also provide a comforting flavor and aid in relaxation.

Ingredients:

- 2 tablespoons dried feverfew
- 1 teaspoon valerian root
- 1 cup of hot water

Instructions:

1. Fill a pot with fresh cold water. Bring the water to a boil.

2. Put 8-10 feverfew flowers in a cup or mug.

3. Pour boiling water over the feverfew flowers. Steep for 3-5 minutes.

4. Add 1 teaspoon of valerian root to the tea. Steep for an additional 5 minutes.

5. Strain the tea and enjoy.

Benefits:

Feverfew contains compounds called parthenolide which can help to block certain cytokines that contribute to migraine pain. Valerian root is known for its calming and soothing effects and can help to relax the body and reduce stress. When combined, this herbal remedy could provide headache relief while calming the mind and body for a more relaxing experience.

Lavender, Rosemary, and Peppermint Oil Infusion

For folks looking for a natural solution to headaches and other mild pain, lavender, rosemary, and peppermint oil infusion is an effective remedy. Not only does this mixture smell wonderful, but it's also full of powerful anti-inflammatory compounds that help reduce the intensity of headache pain. All you need to do is create a simple oil infusion with these three oils and apply it to your forehead. This can provide instantaneous relief, but even better results can be seen over time with regular use. Start exploring holistic home remedies today with this all-natural solution!

Ingredients:

- 2 tablespoons of almond oil
- 5 drops of lavender essential oil
- 4 drops of rosemary essential oil
- 3 drops of peppermint essential oil

Instructions:

1. Pour the almond oil into a glass bottle.

2. Add the lavender, rosemary, and peppermint essential oils to the almond oil. Secure the lid tightly and shake the bottle to mix all ingredients.

3. Make sure your forehead is clean and dry, then apply a few drops of the oil infusion directly onto your skin. Gently massage into the area for maximum effect.

Benefits:

Lavender oil can aid in relaxation and stress relief, while rosemary is known to be an anti-inflammatory agent. Peppermint oil has often been used to combat headaches as it works on stopping pain signals sent to the brain, providing a soothing and cooling sensation. This natural remedy can provide great relief while also being a calming, pleasant experience.

Chamomile-Lemon Balm-Ginger Tea

Ease your headache woes with Chamomile-Lemon Balm-Ginger Tea, a natural yet highly effective remedy. It combines three herbal powers which work together to relax the body, reduce inflammation, improve digestion, and relieve tension-type headaches. These herbs are well known for their calming and therapeutic effects on the body and mind. They provide an additional layer of support that helps restore balance when taken as part of a regular regimen. Studies have shown that drinking this tea reduces the intensity of headache attacks and even prevents them from occurring in the first place. With its light, fluffy texture, pleasant aroma, and amazing taste, Chamomile-Lemon Balm-Ginger Tea is worth trying if you suffer from occasional headaches!

Ingredients:

- 1 teaspoon of chamomile
- 1 teaspoon of lemon balm
- 1 teaspoon of freshly grated ginger

Instructions:

1. Fill a pot with fresh cold water. Bring the water to a boil.
2. Put all three ingredients into a cup or mug.
3. Pour boiling water over the herbs and ginger. Steep for 3-5 minutes.
4. Strain the tea and enjoy!

Benefits:

Chamomile is well-known for its calming and anti-inflammatory properties, making it a great choice for easing headaches. Lemon balm is known to reduce stress, improve digestion, and even prevent future headaches. Ginger not only adds a nice flavor to the tea but is also known for its natural anti-inflammatory and analgesic benefits. Combined, this herbal remedy is a great way to provide relief while also restoring balance in the body.

Garlic, Ginger, and Honey Compound

Garlic, ginger, and honey are a powerful combination when it comes to relieving headaches. As a natural remedy, this compound is gaining more and more attention due to its ability to naturally reduce pain caused by migraines, tension headaches, and sinus headaches. The roots of garlic and ginger reduce an agitated nervous system which in turn helps relieve headache pain. Additionally, the combination of these two ingredients with honey helps soothe inflammation that is often associated with headaches. Its anti-inflammatory properties aid in reducing the swelling that can also be part of the headache cause. Taking regular doses of this compound is a great way to combat headaches without having to reach for harsh drugs or pills all the time.

Ingredients:

- 3 cloves of garlic
- 1 teaspoon of freshly grated ginger
- 2 tablespoons of honey

Instructions:

1. Peel and mince the garlic cloves.

2. Mix the minced garlic, grated ginger, and honey in a bowl until thoroughly combined.

3. Take one teaspoon of this mixture on an empty stomach every morning for the best results.

Benefits:

Garlic has powerful anti-inflammatory and antioxidant properties, while ginger is an effective natural painkiller. Honey helps soothe the throat and provides a bit of sweetness to the mixture. This natural combination is a great way to reduce headache pain without having to rely on over-the-counter drugs that can cause unpleasant side effects. Additionally, it is easy to prepare and regularly used for maximum results.

Cayenne Pepper and Apple Cider Vinegar Remedy

Seeking relief from a nagging headache? Consider trying the cayenne pepper and apple cider vinegar remedy. The combination of cayenne's active ingredient, capsaicin, with the acetic acid in the vinegar soothes the aching head. Drink this mixture slowly to help take your mind off the pain and allow time for the remedy to kick in. Be aware that you may feel some tingling or warmth around your lips and tongue after drinking, but it's completely normal. While not as instant as popping a pill, taking this natural approach can do wonders for relieving your headache without any side effects.

Ingredients:

- 1 teaspoon of cayenne pepper
- 2 tablespoons of apple cider vinegar

Instructions:

1. Mix the cayenne pepper and apple cider vinegar in a glass.

2. Fill the glass with 8 ounces of warm water. Stir until all ingredients are well blended.

3. Drink the mixture slowly, allowing time for it to work its magic.

Benefits:

Cayenne pepper contains capsaicin which works to reduce inflammation and pain. Apple cider vinegar is also known for its anti-inflammatory properties, and it helps to balance the acidity in the body. The combination of these ingredients works to soothe the pain from headaches and provide relief without any harsh side effects. Additionally, this remedy is easy to make and can be used whenever a headache strikes.

Mullein and St. John's Wort Elixir

If you're looking for a natural remedy to your pesky, persistent headaches, then look no further than the powerful combination of passionflower, catnip, and licorice root tea. Holistic healers have used this trio of organic ingredients for years as an effective way to stop head pain in its tracks. Passionflower helps to relax the muscles, while catnip soothes tension in the head and neck. And finally, licorice root serves as an anti-inflammatory agent that reduces any discomfort. Combined in one delicious and easy-to-make tea blend, this incredible remedy is a surefire way to finally achieve lasting headache relief.

Ingredients:

- 1 teaspoon of mullein
- 1 teaspoon of St John's Wort

Instructions:

1. Fill a pot with fresh cold water. Bring the water to a boil.

2. Put both mullein and St John's Wort into a mug or cup.

3. Pour the boiling water over the herbs. Steep for 8-10 minutes.

4. Strain and enjoy your tea!

Benefits:

Mullein has long been used as a natural remedy for headaches due to its anti-inflammatory and calming properties. St John's Wort is also known for its ability to reduce tension and relieve pain. The combination of these two herbs makes for an incredibly effective elixir that can help provide relief to those with chronic headaches. Additionally, this tea blend is easy to make and can be enjoyed daily for maximum effect.

Passionflower, Catnip, and Licorice Root Tea

For those looking for natural relief from headaches, herbal teas are an excellent place to start. Passionflower, catnip, and licorice root tea have been used for centuries as remedies for frequent headaches. Passionflower is believed to provide a calming effect on the body and can even treat anxiety-induced headaches. Catnip has antimicrobial properties that can fight off infections and reduce inflammation. Finally, licorice root has anti-inflammatory and pain-alleviating benefits that make it incredibly effective in treating headache pain. Whatever your herbal tea preference may be, it can probably provide some measure of relief when it comes to managing headaches.

Ingredients:

- 1 teaspoon of passionflower

- 1 teaspoon of catnip

- 1 teaspoon of licorice root

Instructions:

1. Fill a medium-sized saucepan with two cups of cold water.

2. Bring the water to a boil and add all three herbs.

3. Reduce the heat to medium-low and let the mixture simmer for 10 minutes.

4. Strain the tea into a mug and enjoy!

Benefits:

Passionflower is a natural sedative that can help reduce anxiety and tension headaches. Catnip has antimicrobial properties that can fight off infections and reduce inflammation. And licorice root is a natural anti-inflammatory that can help alleviate pain and discomfort. The combination of these three herbs makes for an incredibly soothing and effective tea blend that can provide lasting relief from headaches.

Lemongrass, Rosemary, and Sage Decoction

If your head is pounding and you're too far away from an aspirin bottle, consider trying a lemongrass, rosemary, and sage decoction to help relieve your headache. This home remedy has been used safely by many people over the centuries due to its natural analgesic properties. Once brewed together in hot water, the distinct aroma of these herbal ingredients can transport pain sufferers to a calmer state of mind, providing both physical and emotional relief. Whether you sip it fresh from the stove or cool it down for a refreshing drink, this herbal blend is worth trying out if you're looking for a natural way to treat your headaches.

Ingredients:

- 1 teaspoon of lemongrass
- 2 teaspoons of rosemary
- 1 teaspoon of sage

Instructions:

1. Fill a pot with three cups of cold water and bring it to a boil.

2. Add the lemongrass, rosemary, and sage to the boiling water and reduce the heat to low.

3. Let the herbs steep for 10 minutes, then turn off the heat and strain.

4. Enjoy your decoction, either hot or cold.

Benefits:

Lemongrass is known for its calming and soothing effects, which can reduce stress-induced headaches. Rosemary has anti-inflammatory properties that can help reduce headache pain. Sage is also a natural analgesic and antispasmodic, making it an excellent remedy for headaches.

White Willow Bark Syrup

White willow bark has long been praised for its ability to alleviate headaches, and now that same ease can be found thanks to the introduction of white willow bark syrup! This special syrup is made with a combination of natural herbs that have been proven to provide relief when taken at the onset of a headache. It's also incredibly easy to use; just mix the remedy with water or juice and drink it down. Those looking for fast and effective relief should consider giving this syrup a try; you won't regret the results!

Ingredients:

- 2 tablespoons of white willow bark
- 1 cup of honey

Instructions:

1. In a medium-sized pot, combine the white willow bark and honey.

2. Bring the mixture to a simmer over medium heat, stirring occasionally.

3. Let the syrup reduce for about 20 minutes until it has a thick consistency.

4. Strain the mixture into a glass jar and store it in the refrigerator for up to two weeks.

5. To use, mix 1-2 tablespoons of the syrup with a cup of water or juice and drink.

Benefits:

White willow bark contains salicin, a natural pain reliever that can help reduce the severity of headaches. Honey is also known for its anti-inflammatory properties and can help soothe any throbbing pain. This syrup is a great natural remedy for those looking to find relief from a headache fast!

Turmeric and Coconut Oil Paste

Turmeric and coconut oil paste have long been used to help provide relief from headaches. The combination of these natural ingredients creates a powerful paste that can be applied directly to the head or forehead area to alleviate pain and reduce inflammation. The coconuts contain essential fats that, when mixed with turmeric, have anti-inflammatory properties, while the turmeric itself contains curcumin, an antioxidant that is also known for its natural pain-relieving abilities. Not only do both ingredients provide soothing benefits, but they are also easy to find and prepare. With consistent use, this protective paste could become your go-to when it comes to alleviating headache pain quickly and naturally.

Ingredients:

- 2 tablespoons of turmeric
- 2 tablespoons of coconut oil

Instructions:

1. Mix the turmeric and coconut oil in a small bowl until it forms a thick paste.

2. Apply the paste directly to your forehead or head area, massaging gently.

3. Leave the paste on for 10 minutes, then rinse off with warm water.

4. Repeat the process 2-3 times a day until relief is achieved.

5. Store any remaining paste in the refrigerator for up to one week.

6. Enjoy your newfound relief!

Benefits:

Turmeric is known for its antiseptic, anti-inflammatory, and antioxidant properties, which are all beneficial in alleviating pain. Coconut oil contains essential fatty acids that can also help reduce inflammation and relieve headaches. Together, these two ingredients work to provide a soothing remedy for headache pain.

Tips and Precautions

When using herbal antibiotics to treat headaches, it's crucial to take a few precautions to maximize their effectiveness. Consult with your physician or pharmacist first to determine if they are the best choice and if the medication will interact with any other treatments, you might be taking. Make sure you understand the full dosage and duration of treatment. Never take more than necessary, as it can compromise its efficacy. Try drinking plenty of fluids, eating healthy foods, and getting enough rest since headache remedies often work better when your body is taken care of first. Lastly, do not forget about preventative measures such as stress reduction and good posture, which can help keep headaches at bay in the future. Although these remedies are natural and generally safe, there are a few tips to keep in mind.

- Patch test any of the ingredients before applying them directly to your skin, as some people may have an allergic reaction.

- Try not to use too much of the remedy as this can irritate.

- Keep all remedies stored out of reach of young children and pets.

- Use these remedies as directed to ensure optimal results.

- If you are pregnant, nursing, or have any medical conditions, consult your doctor before using these remedies.

- Drink plenty of water throughout the day as well, as dehydration can lead to headaches in some cases.

- Use any of these remedies as needed, but if your headaches persist or worsen, be sure to seek the advice of a healthcare professional.

- Look for high-quality organic ingredients to ensure the best results.

- Add a few drops of essential oils, such as peppermint or lavender, to any of the remedies for an extra soothing effect.

- Experiment with different recipes to find what works best for you.

- Above all else, enjoy the process and take time out of your day to relax and breathe. This is the best way to reduce stress and keep your headaches at bay!

Herbal remedies have been used to treat headaches for centuries and can still be just as effective today. From licorice root tea to turmeric and coconut oil paste, various herbal remedies can provide natural relief from headache pain. Some of these recipes may take some time to prepare, but the payoff could be worth it if you find yourself searching for a soothing solution. Taking care of your body means understanding what natural remedies can do for you, and herbal solutions have proven themselves time and time again as perfect alternatives to conventional headache treatments. So, the next time your head is pounding, consider turning to nature for a remedy!

Chapter 9

Herbal Antibiotics for Common Ailments

Herbal remedies have withstood the test of time since they've been around for centuries. Many cultures have unique natural medicine systems that take advantage of various plants, roots, and other substances found in nature. They can be used to treat common illnesses like infections and pains and more chronic conditions such as skin issues. When formulated properly, herbal medicines are an effective, safe form of alternative care that can do wonders for our health without the harsh side effects associated with many conventional medications.

With a bit of research, many people find they can make their herbal mixtures at home or purchase them from reliable sources to get the advantages of a centuries-old tradition. This chapter will provide several recipes of herbal antibiotics for common ailments with step-by-step instructions for each one. For each recipe, you'll also find why this combination of natural ingredients helps people feel better. The remedies are divided into three sections: herbal remedies for infection, pain, and skin issues.

Herbal Remedies for Infection

Herbal remedies have been used to treat infections for centuries, with recent research showing that they can be an effective alternative or supplement to traditional treatments. Herbs such as garlic, thyme, and St. John's wort have potent antibacterial and antiviral compounds that can help fight infection quickly and gently. Garlic is especially beneficial because it has antibacterial and antiviral properties, making it an ideal choice for treating various infections. In addition, herbs like licorice root and marshmallows can be useful for soothing inflamed tissues that may accompany an infection. As part of a healthy lifestyle, incorporating herbal remedies into your treatment plan when fighting infections can be incredibly helpful in improving your body's ability to heal itself naturally.

Garlic-Honey Antibiotic

Revered for its healing powers, the garlic-honey antibiotic recipe is said to have first originated in ancient Greece. Considered a natural wonder, this concoction is surprisingly simple and inexpensive to make at home. The resulting syrup can be stored for up to six months and taken as an immune system booster or remedy for symptoms of cold, allergy, or respiratory illness. With its proven antibacterial properties alongside a sweet flavor profile enhanced by fiery notes of garlic, this age-old blend is sure to soothe even the most stubborn of illnesses.

Ingredients:

- 4 cloves of garlic
- 2 tablespoons of honey

balm has antioxidant properties, it can also help to protect against cell damage from free radicals, helping to heal the skin faster.

Herbal remedies have been around for centuries and offer a wide variety of uses, from treating skin issues to helping with digestive problems. From plantain-tamanu cream to lemon balm tea, these natural treatments can provide relief for numerous ailments without the need for harsh chemicals or expensive treatments. Not only do they offer effective solutions to your health concerns, but they also provide additional benefits like reduced inflammation, quicker healing times, and increased protection from environmental damage. Whether you are looking for relief from skin issues or just want to find an all-natural remedy for everyday health problems, herbal antibiotics could be the perfect solution.

Chapter 10

Herbal Antibiotics for Digestion

Herbal antibiotics are a lesser-known yet effective way of helping to remedy digestive issues. Incorporating them into your lifestyle can provide your body with all the critical nutrients necessary for optimal digestion, allowing it to heal naturally and promote healthier gut bacteria, which can protect you against inflammation and other illnesses. Herbal antibiotics have fewer side effects than traditional medication, so they are becoming increasingly popular amongst health-conscious individuals looking for an alternative healing option.

The bonus of using herbal antibiotics is that they offer a holistic approach that looks at the body and its environment as a whole, looking at both dietary and lifestyle choices as important components of well-being. If you've been trying to find a natural solution for your digestive ailments, look no further. This chapter will provide several recipes of herbal antibiotics for digestion with step-by-step instructions for each one. It will also explain why the combination of these ingredients helps people feel better.

Herbal Antibiotic for Digestion

Herbal antibiotics are becoming increasingly popular for addressing digestive issues because of their holistic approach and reduced chance of adverse side effects. Used since ancient times, herbal antibiotics contain natural properties capable of eliminating harmful bacteria while aiding the growth of beneficial gut flora. Prebiotics may also be included to target specific digestion ailments. While herbs alone likely won't be enough to cure an illness, they can significantly reduce symptoms and help restore balance to the body faster than allopathic medicine. As people continue to turn towards more natural alternatives for their health, herbal antibiotics are a viable option for those seeking relief from digestive troubles.

Ingredients:

- 2 tablespoons of ground ginger
- 1 teaspoon of turmeric
- 1/2 teaspoon of fennel seeds
- 1 tablespoon of apple cider vinegar

Instructions:

1. Measure out all the ingredients and place them into a bowl or mortar.

2. Using a pestle, grind the herbs together until they are well combined and a paste is formed.

3. Add the apple cider vinegar and stir together until all ingredients are evenly distributed in the mixture.

4. Take one tablespoon of the herbal antibiotic each day, either directly or mixed into warm water or tea.

Benefits:

Ginger has been used for centuries to treat digestive issues like nausea, vomiting, and abdominal pain. Turmeric has potent antioxidant properties that help scavenge free radicals and protect the body from oxidative damage that inflammatory digestive conditions may cause. Fennel is known for its carminative properties, which helps reduce gas and bloating in the digestive system.

Fennel, Thyme, and Marshmallow Tea

If you're looking for a simple and delicious way to improve your digestion, fennel, thyme, and marshmallow tea is a perfect choice. This herbal blend combines the fragrant flavor of fennel, the herbaceous aroma of thyme, and the soothing effects of marshmallow root that improve gut health. Steeped in hot water, this tea reduces inflammation and fortifies the digestive system by aiding in the digestion and absorption of food. With its pleasant flavor and easy availability, it's an ideal choice for anyone looking to promote their digestive health.

Ingredients:

- 1 teaspoon of dried fennel seed
- 1 teaspoon of dried thyme
- 1 tablespoon of marshmallow root

Instructions:

1. Measure out all the ingredients and place them into a teapot.
2. Fill the teapot with 8 ounces of boiling water.
3. Allow the tea to steep for 10 minutes.
4. Strain the mixture into a cup and enjoy!

Benefits:

Fennel is a natural carminative, meaning it helps reduce gas and bloating in the digestive system. It also has antispasmodic properties that help ease cramping and discomfort associated with the digestive system. The thyme in this tea expels gas from the stomach and intestines and reduces inflammation in the gastrointestinal tract. Marshmallow root is known for its mucilage content, which soothes and coats the entire digestive system, reducing irritation and inflammation. This herbal blend helps to reduce digestive distress while promoting a healthy environment for nutrient absorption.

Turmeric, Ginger and Cinnamon Tea

Drinking a soothing cup of tea made with turmeric, ginger, and cinnamon is an enjoyable way to help support digestion. Turmeric contains curcumin, a powerful anti-inflammatory that has been linked to improvements in digestion problems such as indigestion, nausea, stomach pain, and bloating. Ginger has long been used for its antiemetic properties, which are useful for helping reduce or relieve the symptoms of nausea. Combined with the spicy warmth of cinnamon added for its antioxidant effects, this herbal tea blend can be beneficial for anyone looking for relief from digestive discomfort or flavor. Whether sipped after a meal or simply enjoyed throughout the day, this tasty brew is both comforting and beneficial.

Ingredients:

- 1 teaspoon of turmeric powder
- 1 teaspoon of ground ginger
- 1 teaspoon of cinnamon powder

Instructions:

1. Measure out all the ingredients and place them into a teapot.
2. Fill the teapot with 8 ounces of boiling water.
3. Allow the tea to steep for 10 minutes.
4. Strain the mixture into a cup and enjoy!

Benefits:

Turmeric contains curcumin, which has powerful anti-inflammatory properties that can help reduce inflammation in the digestive system. Ginger is a natural antispasmodic that helps ease cramping and abdominal discomfort associated with digestive issues. Cinnamon can help reduce bloating and gas, as well as provide a boost of antioxidants that protect the digestive system from free radical damage. This combination of herbs provides a warm and comforting drink that soothes the digestive system and helps reduce digestive discomfort.

Coriander, Clove, and Peppermint Tea

Enjoy the delicious combination of coriander, clove, and peppermint teas to stimulate digestion. Not only does this tea blend aid in digestion, but it is also wonderfully flavorful and refreshing. Drinking this tea regularly can help maintain a healthy and balanced GI system. A cup of this magical mix after any meal may provide all the support that your stomach needs!

Ingredients:

- 1 teaspoon of coriander seed

- 1 teaspoon of ground cloves

- 2 teaspoons of peppermint leaves

Instructions:

1. Measure out all the ingredients and place them into a teapot.

2. Fill the teapot with 8 ounces of boiling water.

3. Allow the tea to steep for 10 minutes.

4. Strain the mixture into a cup and enjoy!

Benefits:

Coriander activates digestion by stimulating the production of digestive enzymes. Clove has powerful anti-inflammatory properties that help reduce inflammation in the digestive system. Peppermint is known to relax the stomach muscles and reduce bloating, allowing for easier digestion. The combination of these herbs provides a tasty and beneficial tea that helps relieve digestive discomfort while promoting healthy digestion.

Chamomile and Licorice Tea

If you are looking for a natural remedy for digestive issues, chamomile, and licorice tea may be worth a try. This herbal tea blend is surprisingly easy to make. Simply purchasing dried chamomile and licorice root from your local health-food store will do the trick. Many believe that the combination of these beneficial herbs can stimulate the production of gastric juices to support proper digestion. In addition, its soothing effects can reduce bloating, cramping, and other common digestive complaints. Start by sipping on a cup of this tea after meals to experience its potential effect on improved digestion.

Ingredients:

- 1 teaspoon of chamomile flowers
- 1 teaspoon of licorice root powder

Instructions:

1. Measure out all the ingredients and place them into a teapot.
2. Fill the teapot with 8 ounces of boiling water.
3. Allow the tea to steep for 10 minutes.
4. Strain the mixture into a cup and enjoy!

Benefits:

Chamomile has anti-inflammatory and antispasmodic properties that can soothe the digestive tract and reduce stomach cramps. Licorice root contains glycyrrhizic acid, which has been known to stimulate the production of gastric juices to aid in digestion. This tea blend is a great way to reduce digestive discomfort and promote healthy digestion. Give it a try to experience its potential benefits!

Catnip, Calendula, and Ginger Tea

Catnip, Calendula, and Ginger Tea have been used for centuries to support digestive health. Herbalists believe that this combination of herbal tea helps improve digestion by calming common stomach ailments like gas and bloating. Additionally, researchers claim that Catnip can act as a mild sedative which further supports the body's ability to digest foods properly. The anti-inflammatory properties of both Calendula and Ginger may help reduce discomfort associated with indigestion. Catnip, Calendula, and Ginger Tea may be a perfect choice if you're looking for an herbal remedy to improve your digestion.

Ingredients:

- 1 teaspoon of catnip
- 1 teaspoon of calendula petals
- 1/2 teaspoon of ground ginger

Instructions:

1. Measure out all the ingredients and place them into a teapot.

2. Fill the teapot with 8 ounces of boiling water.

3. Allow the tea to steep for 10 minutes.

4. Strain the mixture into a cup and enjoy!

Benefits:

Catnip helps to soothe the stomach and stimulate digestion. Calendula has antiparasitic and anti-inflammatory properties that may reduce digestive discomfort. Ginger helps to calm the digestive system, reduce inflammation, and improve the absorption of food in the intestines. The combination of these herbs makes a strong tea that can help reduce common digestive issues and promote healthy digestion. Give it a try to experience its potential effects!

Tulsi and Cinnamon Tea

Tulsi, or holy basil, is widely regarded for its healing properties that can benefit people's overall health, particularly with digestive issues. In combination with cinnamon tea, many herbalists are effusive in their promotion of the remedy's effect on digestion. In India, especially in traditional Ayurvedic medicine practices, tulsi, and cinnamon tea are recommended to treat indigestion and nausea. The tea can also help reduce the symptoms of irritable bowel syndrome or IBS. With warm water as the base and adding a few leaves of fresh tulsi and a couple of pieces of cinnamon bark boiled together into it, this kind of infusion has not only immense healing benefits but also tastes delicious, being subtly aromatic and warming to the soul.

Ingredients:

- 2 tablespoons of tulsi leaves

- 3 pieces of cinnamon bark

Instructions:

1. Measure out all the ingredients and place them into a teapot.

2. Fill the teapot with 8 ounces of boiling water.

3. Allow the tea to steep for 10 minutes.

4. Strain the mixture into a cup and enjoy!

Benefits:

Tulsi is known to soothe and balance the digestive system, reduce gas and bloating, support the elimination of toxins, and alleviate common symptoms associated with indigestion. Cinnamon has antifungal and antiviral properties, helping to reduce common stomach viruses and infections. This tea blend is a great way to support digestion and promote healthy digestion. Give it a try to experience its potential benefits!

Burdock and Green Tea

Burdock and green tea are both fantastic tools for aiding digestion. Burdock cleanses toxins from your body, such as those found in processed foods, while also helping flush out salt, water, and excess fat. Green tea has many health-boosting properties, like being a natural stimulant and fighting bacteria. It's packed with antioxidants that help speed digestion while protecting the body from damage caused by free radicals. Together, these two herbal medicines offer an effective combination that can support your overall Digestive health and improve your quality of life.

Ingredients:

- 1 teaspoon of dried burdock root

- 2 teaspoons of green tea leaves

Instructions:

1. Measure out all the ingredients and place them into a teapot.

2. Fill the teapot with 8 ounces of boiling water.

3. Allow the tea to steep for 10 minutes.

4. Strain the mixture into a cup and enjoy!

Benefits:

Burdock has antimicrobial, antiviral, and antifungal properties that cleanse the digestive system of toxins. It also flushes out excess water, fat, and salt from the body. Green tea is packed with antioxidants that help to speed up digestion while also protecting the body from damage caused by free radicals. The combination of these two herbs makes a strong and effective tea that helps to improve overall Digestive health. Try it out and experience its potential benefits!

Herbal antibiotics can be used as natural remedies to help promote healthy digestion and reduce common digestive issues. From tulsi and cinnamon tea to burdock and green tea, many different herbal teas can be brewed at home with simple ingredients. Each tea blend has its unique benefits and medicinal properties. Try out some of these recipes to see how they can help improve your digestive health and overall well-being.

Conclusion

Herbal antibiotics are quickly becoming the go-to choice for many people's health care needs. They offer an alternative to traditional antibiotics and make it possible to gain control over daily problems without resorting to dangerous drugs. However, it is essential to fully understand how herbal antibiotics work before using them. Most of these products contain natural ingredients that can heal and protect the body in its fight against disease, but it is still crucial to read all instructions carefully and follow the recommended dosage. Additionally, it can be beneficial to talk with a trusted healthcare professional about the best usage for any given product or condition.

There are many different kinds of herbal antibiotics, each one with its own unique set of ingredients and intended purposes. Systemic antibiotics are meant to treat infections throughout the body and are usually taken orally. Non-systemic antibiotics are meant to treat localized areas, such as a sore throat or ear infection, and can be applied topically or taken orally. Synergist antibiotics are used in combination with other treatments to increase their effectiveness, such as when taking them with an herbal tea or tincture.

Once you have chosen which type of product is right for your needs, it is important to consider how to prepare it properly. Building your herbal lab can be a great way to ensure that you are getting the highest quality ingredients in their purest form. You can find kits online or in health stores that have everything you need. Additionally, there are many safety tips and tricks to keep in mind during the preparation process.

When harvesting herbs for use in your herbal lab, there are also some tips and tricks to keep in mind. Knowing the optimal time to begin harvesting, how to properly dry the herbs, and which parts of the plant are most beneficial can help you get the most out of your product.

This guide is an invaluable resource for anyone looking to make herbal antibiotics. It covered detailed information on the different kinds of herbs, the properties of each, and their intended uses. Additionally, it is filled with tips and tricks on how to properly prepare and store your product for the best results.

Finally, it is essential to understand the various herbal antibiotics available for specific ailments. Herbal antibiotics can be incredibly helpful for headaches, common ailments such as colds and flu, and digestive issues. As always, it is crucial to read all instructions carefully so that you can get the most out of your product and have a successful experience with herbal antibiotics.

By understanding the different types of herbal antibiotics available and getting familiar with the preparation process, you will be well prepared to use these products for your healthcare needs. With this knowledge, you can make educated decisions on the best ways to use herbal antibiotics and have a successful experience with these natural remedies.

Thank you for buying and reading/listening to our book. If you found this book useful/helpful please take a few minutes and leave a review on Amazon.com or Audible.com (if you bought the audio version).

References

(N.d.-a). Researchgate.net. https://www.researchgate.net/publication/349088594_Herbal_antibiotics_A_Review

(N.d.-b). Nih.gov. https://www.ncbi.nlm.nih.gov/pmc/articles/PMC7767362/

(N.d.-c). Mdlinx.com. https://www.mdlinx.com/article/hold-the-prescription-try-these-7-natural-antibiotics-instead/j6m1ie8J4JmSrMCbMbAJk

7 best natural antibiotics: Uses, evidence, and effectiveness. (2020, January 1). Medicalnewstoday.com. https://www.medicalnewstoday.com/articles/321108

Brusie, C. (2016, November 23). What are the most effective natural antibiotics? Healthline. https://www.healthline.com/health/natural-antibiotics

Feel Good, Family. (n.d.). Natural antibiotics to stockpile now: 10 herbs and foods that kill superbugs. feelgoodfamily.cz. https://www.feelgoodfamily.cz/natural-antibiotics-to-stockpile-now--10-herbs-and-foods-that-kill-superbugs/

Herbal antibiotics: Fighting infections naturally. (1 C.E., January 1). Good Health. https://www.goodhealth.co.nz/health-articles/article/herbal-antibiotics-fighting-infections-naturally

Sjoberg, V., & Ac., L. (2019, September 29). 8 effective, natural antibiotics to help beat infections. Chopra. https://chopra.com/articles/8-effective-natural-antibiotics-to-help-beat-infections

Milton Keynes UK
Ingram Content Group UK Ltd.
UKHW020630031023
429856UK00015B/598